A Study of
Brief Psychotherapy

A Study of
Brief Psychotherapy

D. H. MALAN
Tavistock Clinic, London

A PLENUM/ROSETTA EDITION

Library of Congress Cataloging in Publication Data

Malan, David Huntingford.
    A study of brief psychotherapy.

    "A Plenum/Rosetta edition."
    Reprint of the ed. published by Tavistock Publications, London, and Thomas,
Springfield, Ill., which was issued as no. 8 of Mind & medicine monographs.
    Bibliography: p.
    Includes index.
    1. Psychotherapy. I. Title. II. Series: Mind & medicine monographs; 8.
[RC480.5.M32 1975]   616.8'914   75-30916
ISBN 0-306-20019-8

First paperback printing 1975

© D. H. Malan, 1963

A Plenum/Rosetta Edition
Published by Plenum Publishing Corporation
227 West 17th Street, New York, N.Y. 10011

United Kingdom edition published by Plenum Press, London
A Division of Plenum Publishing Company, Ltd.
Davis House (4th Floor), 8 Scrubs Lane, Harlesden, London, NW10 6SE, England

Printed in the United States of America

Summary

The original aim of the present work, which was initiated by Dr. Michael Balint, was to explore Brief Psychotherapy carried out by psycho-analysts who are relatively skilled and experienced. To this has been added an attempt to reconcile the 'clinical' and 'objective' approaches to psychodynamic material, by treating clinical judgements exactly as rigorously as is appropriate, no more and no less.

A review of previous work leads to little definite conclusion. A complete spectrum of views can be found, from the most 'conservative' (e.g. brief psychotherapy is only effective in the mildest and most recent illnesses; the technique used should be superficial—any attempt to go 'deeper' will lead to long-term therapy; and the results are only palliative) to the most 'radical' (seriously ill patients can be extensively helped by a technique containing most of the essential elements of long-term methods such as psycho-analysis).

The present work is based essentially on the therapies of nineteen patients, treated by a team of therapists under the leadership of Dr. Balint. The study is largely retrospective, but it is designed to fill some of the important gaps to be found in the literature:

1. Detailed case histories are given of all patients treated;
2. Particular attention is paid to long follow-up;
3. A method of assessing therapeutic results has been developed which is regarded as psychodynamically valid and is based on published evidence;
4. The relation is examined between outcome and
   (a) the characteristics of patients,
   (b) the characteristics of technique.

The methods used are clinical or statistical, where appropriate, and for (b) include a quantitative analysis of the case records, which were dictated from memory. It is shown that clinical judgement and quantitative analysis often support each other.

Summary

The results are as follows:

1. The widely held conservative view that it is the 'mild' illnesses of recent onset that are the most suitable for brief psychotherapy is not supported.
2. On the contrary, there is strong evidence that other factors are more important, and that quite far-reaching and lasting improvements can be obtained in relatively severe and long-standing illnesses.
3. The cumulative evidence is very strong that (a) interpretation of the transference in general, and (b) interpretation of the link between transference feelings and the relation to parents in particular, not only carried few dangers in these therapies, but also played a very important part in leading to a favourable outcome.

In short, the results of our work consistently support the radical rather than the conservative view.

It is finally shown that, in almost all the hypotheses reached, a single unifying factor can be found. It is suggested that this may be one of the important 'non-specific' factors common to many forms of psychotherapy.

The reader is referred particularly to Chapter 12, pp. 268–72, for a critical discussion of the quality of the evidence.

To Dr. Michael Balint
Mentor, and opponent in many controversies

Mrs. Enid Balint
and all members of the Workshop, especially the final members
and all most closely involved in the work reported here:

Mr. J. L. Boreham
Dr. R. H. Gosling
Dr. J. J. M. Jacobs
Dr. Agnes Main
Dr. T. F. Main
Dr. M. Pines
Mr. E. H. Rayner
Dr. J. L. Rowley

CONTENTS

ix

Contents

LIST OF TABLES

ACKNOWLEDGEMENTS

My grateful thanks are due to:

Dr. A. R. Jonckheere of the Department of Psychology, University College, London, for his constant patience in advising me on statistical problems.

Mr. E. H. Rayner, for his help over the dreary task of checking some of my clinical judgements.

Miss Olive Plowman, whose patience and willingness for hard work have made the final preparation of this book—for me—so easy.

Our appreciation is also due to all the secretaries who carried out the seemingly impossible task of taking down our discussions in shorthand and making sense out of them afterwards: Miss Doris Young, Miss Valerie Hume, Miss Ann Gatland, Miss Molly Curran, and Mrs. Adelaide Blunden; and to Mrs. Kathleen Clare of the Ellesmere Secretarial Bureau, Fleet, Hants., for her accurate typing of six extra copies of the manuscript.

PART I

HISTORICAL AND THEORETICAL SURVEY

CHAPTER 1

Introductory

In spite of the immense advances of the present century in the understanding and treatment of neurotic illness, many problems remain that are both pressing and largely unsolved. The present work approaches two of these: first, that of reducing the length of psychotherapy; and second, that of basing generalizations about psychotherapy on evidence that is publishable and also contains the minimum of unsupported inference. The value of any contribution, however small, to these two problems needs little emphasis.

The book consists of a study of the clinical work carried out by a team of psycho-analysts, of which the author was a member, under the leadership of Dr. Michael Balint. The work was originated by Balint and arose from his recognition that however favourably 'long-term' psychotherapy—and particularly psychoanalysis—may influence the lives of selected individuals, in comparison with the amount of neurotic unhappiness in the world its contribution can never be anything but negligible. He has therefore turned in the last few years to investigating how the experience of a lifetime of psycho-analysis may contribute towards therapeutic aims which are more limited but of wider application. His book, *The Doctor, his Patient and the Illness* (1957), was the result of applying this idea to psychotherapy in general practice. There the therapeutic work is relatively superficial and is carried out by general practitioners with relatively little training. The present research is complementary to this. The aim has been to investigate brief psychotherapy carried out, on a much 'deeper' and more intense level, by therapists with a fairly complete knowledge and experience of the technique of psycho-analysis. Although such work has of course been done before, it has led to no systematic body of knowledge and to little that is generally agreed; so that no apology is needed for a wish to approach the subject once more with an open mind and from the very beginning.

3

All members of the team have contributed to the thinking set out here, and particularly to the formulation of hypotheses. My own contribution has been the testing of these hypotheses, and the search for new ones, in the data provided by those cases— about twenty—treated in the first two years of the work. It is necessary to state that I do not necessarily speak for the team as a whole. The methods used are entirely my own responsibility; and the conclusions reached are not necessarily acceptable to the other members—though deriving much from them, and I hope representing a systematic exploration in the directions in which their own thought has been leading.

The undertaking of this work has led to the second of the two main problems, that of handling data on psychotherapy in such a way that hypotheses or conclusions are based on something more than 'clinical impression', and of presenting the evidence in such a way that it can be judged, to some extent at least, by an independent observer. This second, 'methodological' problem has seemed in the past hardly less intractable than the purely therapeutic problem. The literature on psychotherapy shows the usual divergence between 'subjective' methods, which depend on apparently unverifiable inference, and methods which, the more 'objective' they are, the more clinically meaningless they become. Yet, growing experience has led me—and an increasing number of other authors—ever more certainly to the conclusion that this divergence is at least partly artificial, and is maintained by emotional problems rooted in the traditions of psycho-analysis and experimental psychology. Much effort has therefore been given to reducing the divergence by trying to treat clinical judgements in exactly as rigorous a manner as is appropriate, no more and no less.

The attempt to apply rigorous methods meets very serious difficulties caused by the main orientation of the work and the conditions in which it was undertaken. The orientation was essentially clinical and exploratory, and all members of the team were motivated more by clinical enthusiasm than by any desire to subject themselves to the discipline necessary for the thorough testing of scientific hypotheses. Moreover, since there was no financial support, all therapists and secretaries had to work in such time as could be spared from heavy routine commitments. This research, therefore, suffers from serious defects: clinical records dictated from memory, and retrospective judgements only partially checked by independent observers. For this reason the main emphasis must be essentially clinical; but particular atten-

4

tion is given to the publication of the evidence on which judgements are based, to the presence or absence of 'controls', to the
need to explore fallacies, and to the possibility of obtaining a
given result by chance alone. In addition, more 'objective' methods
are explored in an attempt to reduce—though far from eliminate—
the subjective and unverifiable element in the evidence presented.

It is shown that, in spite of the deficiencies in the material, the
clinical and the more 'obejctive' approaches often point in the same
direction. In the hands of a single observer, this must obviously be
treated with reserve. Nevertheless, the final result is a series of
hypotheses which—though each alone is derived from inconclusive evidence—support each other by making sense as a whole,
and are in turn supported by principles established independently,
namely those by now well accepted for psycho-analysis itself.
This kind of convergence of evidence is often all that is possible in
scientific problems of many different kinds. I should like to refer
the reader especially to a critical discussion of the status of the
evidence (pages 268–72). And finally, there emerge certain incontrovertible facts which—though indeed reported in the literature before—have never been widely accepted, and which could be
of considerable practical value in the future.

There follows a long exposition of the background to this work,
all of which is necessary if the problems involved in brief psychotherapy are to be fully understood, and if the present position
reached is to be seen clearly in its historical setting.

CHAPTER 2

Historical Approach

THE HISTORY OF PSYCHO-ANALYSIS

The evolution of psycho-analysis may be regarded as an 'ecological' process involving the interaction of patients of a particular kind and therapists of a particular outlook, within the environment of Western civilization. When any such process begins, there will usually be seen a tendency towards change in some definite direction, leading eventually to a state of equilibrium. With psycho-analysis the most easily identified tendency, manifested repeatedly as each new advance was made, has been towards an *increase in the length of therapy*. Thus anyone who tries to develop a technique of brief psychotherapy is trying to reverse an evolutionary process impelled by powerful forces, and it is as well that he should first identify these forces, and specifically try to oppose them.

The history of psycho-analysis, regarded from this point of view, may be summarized as follows (see Breuer and Freud, 1895; Freud, 1896, 1904, and 1914). The original observation, made by Breuer, was that hysterical symptoms could be relieved by making the patient re-live, under hypnosis, painful memories and feelings that had been forgotten ('repressed'). Freud, finding that not all patients could be hypnotized, replaced this method by suggesting forcefully to the patient in the waking state that there were things that she had forgotten and could remember. He now found, however, that suggestion was often insufficient to overcome a marked *resistance* put up by the patient against recovering these memories. He was able to by-pass this difficulty when he found that, if he simply asked the patient to say what came into her mind in connection with her symptoms, the memories returned in a disguised and symbolized form; and that when he learned how to translate the disguise the memories returned undisguised. With more experience he began to realize that whatever came into the patient's mind (not necessarily in connection with her symptoms) had a bearing on the memories or on the resistance against them; and he concentrated on the latter, finding that when the resistances were pointed out the memories could be recovered without any forcing. In this sequence, from hypnosis through suggestion to 'free association', the tendency for the therapist to become *increasingly passive* is clearly to be observed.

During this time a quite unexpected phenomenon had appeared, namely that patients inevitably began to have intense feelings (*transference*) about the therapist. This was already present in the first case treated by Breuer ('Anna O.'; see Jones, 1953, p. 246) and was the cause of Breuer's abandoning this work altogether. Freud found that, if he interpreted to the patient that these feelings were really not about the therapist at all, but were transferred onto him from some important person in the patient's childhood, then they could be handled without jeopardizing the therapy and could finally be resolved.

Yet there was always present the tendency for each new technique, initially successful, to become less and less reliable. Whereas early patients seemed to be cured through the recovery of comparatively recent memories and the interpretation of the related transference feelings, later patients tended to relapse again and could be cured only by uncovering further memories and transference feelings belonging to increasingly *early childhood*. Analyses were prolonged by two further phenomena: the fact that a single symptom was usually found to have its roots in many quite separate memories and feelings, each of which had to be uncovered before the symptom could be relieved (*over-determination*); and the fact that each root often had to be uncovered many times in different contexts, and not once for all, before relief was permanent (necessity for *working through*).

It became recognized that early relief of symptoms was often simply due to the satisfaction of the patient's need for love provided by the analytical situation ('transference cure'); and that the relapse that frequently occurred at threat of termination could be reversed only by interpreting the patient's anger (*negative transference*) at being abandoned, and relating this to its true source in childhood. Meanwhile the importance of transference has steadily increased. The following is now a standard pattern for an analysis: there is an initial period in which both transference and non-transference interpretations seem to be effective and everything seems to be going well (the 'analytic honeymoon'); there is then a period of resistance in which insight is often lost

7

and interpretations which were previously effective become useless; and finally there develops a state known as the *transference neurosis* in which the patient's whole neurosis is expressed in his relation to the therapist, on whom he often becomes extremely *dependent*. Now, to a large extent, only transference interpretations are of any value; and only after this transference has been interpreted again and again, and related to its true source in childhood, can the situation be resolved.

In the meantime emphasis has gradually shifted. The transference has come to be regarded not as a necessary evil, but as the main therapeutic tool—thus transference is welcomed, and especially negative transference, since the patient's unconscious hatred is felt to be a powerful source of neurosis; memories, especially those concerned with sexual traumata, are regarded as of less importance, and emphasis is now laid on the repetition of neurotic childhood patterns in the relation to the therapist, and the gradual acquisition of insight into these; and finally it is held that one of the most important factors is not so much the insight itself, as the *actual experience* of a new kind of relationship with the therapist, through which these neurotic patterns can be corrected (see Ferenczi and Rank, 1925, p. 59; Alexander and French, 1946, p. 22; Alexander, 1957, p. 71).

Factors leading to longer analyses ('lengthening factors') may be summarized thus:

1. Resistance,
2. Over-determination,
3. Necessity for working through,
4. Roots of neurosis in early childhood,
5. Transference,
6. Dependence,
7. Negative transference connected with termination,
8. The transference neurosis.

At the same time, the ecological view of the history of psychoanalysis makes clear that the list of lengthening factors given above shows only part of the picture, for it contains only those factors to be found in the patient. It is clear that some of the tendency towards long analyses may well be due to factors in the analyst, of which we may list the following:

9. A tendency towards passivity and the willingness to follow where the patient leads,
10. The 'sense of timelessness' (Stone, 1951) conveyed to the patient,

8

11. Therapeutic perfectionism,
12. The increasing preoccupation with ever deeper and earlier experiences.

The result of all these factors has been that, whereas early analyses tended to last a few months, nowadays an analysis that lasts twice as many years is nothing remarkable.

It is clear that a rationally based technique of brief psychotherapy must be based on a conscious opposition to one or more of these factors, particularly those in the therapist. Moreover, since different workers have regarded different factors as of prime importance, this list provides a good frame of reference within which the different kinds of technique may be considered.

THE CHARACTERISTICS OF THE EARLY SHORT ANALYSES, WITH SPECIAL REFERENCE TO THERAPEUTIC RESULTS

Although almost all of the lengthening factors mentioned in the previous section, if undesirable, are perfectly intelligible, there is one that remains a mystery. This is not so much that each new technique is eventually proved unreliable, as that before this happens it apparently gives good results. The therapeutic currency, so to speak, is subject to a continuous process of depreciation or inflation.

In confirmation of this, Balint has often remarked that case histories of apparently successful short analyses occur quite frequently in the early literature and then seem to disappear completely. This undocumented observation may be confirmed by a study of the German psycho-analytic journals published between 1909 and 1920, although a complication is introduced by the fact that after 1914, because of the war, the volume of the literature markedly declines. In fact, case histories in which improvement was definitely claimed are not as common as might be supposed—I found only seven[1] in the years 1909–1914—but it is also true that in the years 1915–1920 I succeeded in finding none. On the face of it, therefore, the early analysts seem to have possessed the secret of brief psychotherapy, and with increasing experience to have lost it.

The resolution of this apparent paradox which immediately comes to mind is that these early successes were merely 'transference cures', and that longer follow-up would have proved them illusory. We know, for instance, that the first case of all, Anna O.,

---

[1] Apart from the two shown in *Table 1* (p. 11), these are: Brill (1910), Wulff (1910), Dattner (1911), Benni (1911), and Stekel (1911). In the last two there is the implication, but no specific statement, of improvement.

claimed by Breuer to have 'regained her mental balance entirely' (Breuer and Freud, 1895), later became 'quite unhinged' (see Jones, 1953, p. 247), though it is also true that she eventually recovered and led an extremely useful life.

Yet such information as we have on these early cases does not support the view that they all relapsed—though it is of course impossible to distinguish between permanent improvements due to therapy and the kind of 'spontaneous' improvements for which there is so much recent evidence (see Chapter 7, pp. 151–62). Thus among those treated by Freud:

1. Dora (Freud, 1905), a hysterical patient treated for eleven weeks in 1900, was seen for a single session fifteen months later. She had been much better, but had recently developed a facial neuralgia which Freud was able to interpret as due to transference feelings. Finally, Freud writes: 'Years have gone by since her visit. In the meantime the girl has married . . .' and the implication is that she remained well.

2. The 'Rat Man' (Freud, 1909), a severe obsessional treated for eleven months in 1907, was apparently completely cured. Jones (1955, p. 294) writes: 'The result was brilliant and the patient was very successful in his life and work. Unfortunately he was killed during the first world war.'

Moreover, among the seven 'successful' cases in the early German literature treated by analysts other than Freud, there are two specifically stated to have been followed up for two years or more. The details are shown in *Table 1*.

Finally, chance has put into our hands three patients who have been followed up for exceptional lengths of time. The first two are reported by Oberndorf (1947):

1. A woman of 35 treated in 1909 for depression, intense anxiety, and terrifying hallucinations. She was seen twice a week for a year, recovered from her symptoms, and (in 1947) had written to Oberndorf once a year ever since to say that she was still well—a continuous follow-up of thirty-seven years.

2. A man of 27 seen in 1913 for claustrophobia and a severe conflict over sex. He recovered from the claustrophobia after a year's treatment and two years later was still well, though at that time he had chosen to solve his sexual conflict by abstinence. Later, however, he married and raised a family. Thirty-two years later (1945) he consulted Oberndorf again, having become depressed

TABLE 1 CASES SUCCESSFULLY TREATED BY EARLY ANALYSTS AND FOLLOWED UP FOR 2 TO 3 YEARS

Reference	Patient Sex	Age	Complaint	Length of treatment	Result	Follow-up
Binswanger (1912)	F	20	Phobia of boots, attacks of constipation, 15 years.	'178 days', presumably about 6/12.	Phobia disappeared; constipation improved but still present.	6/12, 2 years
Tannenbaum (1913)	F	23	Abdominal pain, dyspareunia, anxiety, depression.	? 8 weeks 'Frequent visits.'	'Excellent health.'	3 years

because of waning potency, but until that time he had remained symptom-free.

3. The best documented of all these cases, however, is a man of 25 treated by Eder (1911). His complicated symptoms included pain in his neck, inability to eat among strangers, a great dislike of washing, and severe sexual inhibition. Eder saw him once or twice a week for about three months (i.e. twenty-five to thirty sessions) and states that his pain had gone, he was able to eat in restaurants, and he was able to wash, but that he still felt it was 'finer not to have sexual intercourse'. This patient was rediscovered by chance forty-two years later (Hunter and MacAlpine, 1953). It is clear that Eder was somewhat optimistic in his original assessment—for example, for many years the patient had been very reluctant to eat in public. Nevertheless, although he had never married, he had lived 'a not unhappy, if isolated, restricted, and often troubled existence . . . and he remained well enough never to miss a day's work'—until 1951, when he made a suicidal attempt. The extraordinary sequel to this is that he then became quite symptom-free and has remained so until recently (Hunter, personal communication, 1957).

Thus the disappearance of these successful short analyses from the literature cannot be entirely explained away by the suggestion that their therapeutic effects were all illusory, and the mystery remains.

That the loss of therapeutic efficiency that apparently occurred later was due at least partly to some kind of inflation, and not simply (for instance) to a change in the kind of patient treated, is indicated by the fact that in 1909–1914 the early analysts were achieving these therapeutic results with a technique closely resembling that which Freud had already abandoned ten or fifteen years before. This technique had certain characteristics to which we may give the name 'primitive': the analyst was very *active* and paid little or no attention either to *resistance* or to *transference*—and this at a time when Freud (1912) was already writing of the transference as 'inevitable' and discussing at length how it was used by the patient as resistance. Not only this, but the atmosphere and subject-matter of the analyses also had certain primitive characteristics: work was extremely *dramatic* and often culminated in the confession of some *traumatic sexual experience*. All these characteristics gradually disappeared after 1914.

A possible explanation for this whole perplexing set of facts is suggested in an observation which has been made by many analysts, including Balint (personal communication) and Edward Glover (much quoted personal communication). This is that even nowadays individual analysts find that their work is subject to the same kind of inflation—they seem often to achieve a few dramatic quick successes early in their careers, and then apparently can never repeat them. It is as if the ontogeny of individual analysts recapitulates the phylogeny of psycho-analysis itself. The only possible explanation (Balint, personal communication; also Watterson, 1960) seems to lie in changes in the *therapist's enthusiasm*. Perhaps the intense interest of any worker new to this field engenders a corresponding heightened excitement in the patient, with the result that repressed feelings come easily to the surface and are experienced with such intensity and completeness that no further working through is necessary. Subsequently this excitement can never quite be recaptured, nor can its effects. This may even partly account in some way for the prevalence in the material of traumatic experiences—those moments in our lives in which so many feelings, already present, are suddenly concentrated and crystallized by some external circumstance. As will be seen, the present work provides some slight but very interesting evidence on this whole question (see pp. 213–14 below).

These considerations add yet another possible lengthening factor, namely *waning enthusiasm*, to the list already given—one that may not be so easily opposed by any conscious effort.

ATTEMPTS TO SHORTEN PSYCHO-ANALYSIS: FERENCZI

After the tremendous initial enthusiasm, there developed during the 1920s considerable pessimism about the growing length and decreasing therapeutic effectiveness of psycho-analysis (see Thompson, 1952, p. 172), and attempts at halting these tendencies were made by some of Freud's collaborators. Chief of these and the only one considered here was Ferenczi, who published his work in a series of papers (e.g. Ferenczi, 1920), and in a book written with Rank (Ferenczi and Rank, 1923, 1925).

Ferenczi's technique was largely based on a conscious opposition to *passivity*, which of all the lengthening factors is the most widely recognized and the most easily opposed. 'Activity'—in one form or another—is thus common to most techniques of brief psychotherapy. The chief active devices that he employed were:

1. Playing a definite role in relation to the patient, of a kind intended to bring out more intensely the patient's neurotic reactions in the form of transference.

2. Setting a time limit to treatment (used previously by Freud, 1918, in the case of the 'Wolf Man', whose therapy was terminated in 1914).
3. Asking the patient to make up phantasies on certain chosen themes ('forced phantasies').
4. Deliberately increasing frustration in the patient by directing him to do, or not to do, certain things (later, asking him to impose these directions on himself); e.g. for an obsessional, not to carry out his rituals.

These devices seem to have been affected by exactly the same process of inflation as were so many other innovations in psycho-analytic technique—they produced some early successes, and then became increasingly unreliable (e.g. see Ferenczi, 1925). Ferenczi himself finally abandoned them. Nowadays such attempts to shorten analysis are rarely reported by orthodox analysts—an exception is the work of Alexander and French, to be considered in Chapter 3—and the increase in the length of analyses has been generally accepted as inevitable.

Thus this whole history emphasizes that anyone who attempts to develop a technique of brief psychotherapy faces the danger of repeating the experience of Freud and the early analysts, and of simply rediscovering in the end the technique of psycho-analysis itself.

Review of Previous Work on Brief Psychotherapy

INTRODUCTION

Apart from the obvious questions of whether brief psychotherapy is possible at all and the length of treatment required, there are three main questions that any work in this field must be designed to answer:

1. *Selection criteria*: Which patients are suitable, and how is it possible to recognize them?
2. *Technique*: What technique should be used?
3. *Outcome*: What kinds of therapeutic result can be achieved?

As will be repeatedly demonstrated in the following pages, these three questions are closely interrelated, and can really only be separated artificially.

A study of the literature soon reveals that the answers given by different workers to these questions are, at the extreme, completely contradictory. Further study makes clear that all these answers can be reduced essentially to the answer to a single question, namely the degree to which brief psychotherapy resembles or differs from more ambitious, more 'radical' long-term methods. We may thus call the extremes the 'conservative' and the 'radical' views respectively. On almost every question both extremes may be found, together with most positions on the spectrum in between. The answers given may be summarized as in *Table 2*.

Thus the very diversity and contradictory nature of the views expressed may be used as a framework within which the whole of the literature on this complex subject may be considered.

THE QUALITY OF THE EVIDENCE

In spite of all these contradictory opinions, it might be supposed that tentative conclusions about various hypotheses would be

15

TABLE 2 SUMMARY OF THE CONSERVATIVE AND
RADICAL VIEWS

Question	Conservative view	Radical view
Selection criteria	Only acute illnesses in basically well-adjusted personalities are suitable. Brief methods should be used only when long-term methods are not available for practical reasons.	Good results can often be achieved in severe, long-standing illnesses. Brief methods have their own positive indications, and may in certain cases be more suitable than long-term methods.
Technique	Interpretations should be kept at a relatively superficial level; dreams, transference, and the childhood origins of neurosis should be avoided.	There is no essential difference between brief and long-term methods, which lie on a continuum. Dreams, transference, and the childhood origins of neurosis may be interpreted freely where appropriate, and may play an essential part in therapy.
Outcome	Results are essentially palliative and consist of 'symptom removal' only. Deeper changes should not be attempted, and can be brought about only by long-term methods.	There is no essential difference between the therapeutic results of brief and long-term methods. Quite far-reaching changes are often possible.

attainable from a careful study of the literature. This is not really so. For one reason or another, the quality of the evidence is always doubtful. At one end of the scale, opinions based on unsupported clinical impression simply cannot be assessed at all. At the other end, there are many statistical studies, some on large numbers of patients, in none of which is the evidence entirely free from objection. Some of these studies, for instance, contain a simple statistical fallacy: that of accepting at face value a figure for the 'significance' of an individual factor in an exploratory study in which a number of different factors were considered—whereas, of course, the more factors that are considered the greater the probability of finding at least one that would have appeared significant in isolation, by chance alone. These authors deserve sympathy, because the temptation to fall into this error is great; but, as has been amply demonstrated, this criticism is no mere statistical sophistry. When attempts have been made to cross-validate such a factor, that is to test it out on a second sample of patients, the result has only too often proved negative—see, for selection criteria, the comprehensive review by Windle (1952), and the paper by Sullivan, Miller, and Smelser (1958), which may be quoted:

'Cross-validation of findings is essential in this area of research. An unexpectedly large proportion of the obtained "significant" differences may vanish on repetition with successive patient groups in the same setting. It seems wise, therefore, to regard findings until they have been cross-validated as only interesting, possibly chance findings which need to be further tested.'

It can hardly be too strongly emphasized that exactly the same attitude has to be adopted to the results reported in the present work.

Even when fallacies of this kind are absent, however, two fundamental difficulties usually remain. The first is that results valid for one kind of technique, therapist, or patient are not necessarily valid for other kinds. The second is one of the major unsolved problems in this whole field, that of finding a valid and reproducible method of assessing therapeutic results. Often the information about the method of assessment used is inadequate; or if it is adequate then the method itself, when considered psychodynamically, is of doubtful validity.

In my opinion, therefore, little of value has so far been demonstrated; but, on the other hand, there are many interesting indications which are highly relevant to the present work.

SELECTION CRITERIA AND THERAPEUTIC RESULTS

Selection criteria can be arranged in a series: at one end, those independent of the type of illness (e.g. acuteness); in the centre, those clearly correlated with the type of illness (e.g. severity of the psychopathology); and, at the other end, those that consist simply of a description of the illness (e.g. acute anxiety states). Since the type of illness automatically fixes the kind of therapeutic result desired, selection criteria and results are best considered together.

17

TABLE 3 OPINIONS IN FAVOUR OF 'HYPOTHESIS A'

Reference	1 Type of patient 2 Type of therapy 3 No. of patients	Kind of evidence or criteria used	Good prognosis	Poor prognosis
Knight (1937)	1 Neurotic 2 Analytically based 3 —	Clinical experience	Recently developed anxieties, obsessions, disabilities, inhibitions.	
Fuerst (1938)	1 Neurotic 2 Analytically based 3 —	Clinical experience	Acute psychogenic symptoms of a hysterical type; acute anxiety or depressive states of a neurotic nature.	Compulsive characters, sexual perversions, homosexuality, disturbances of long duration which influence the whole life situation.
Berliner (1941)	1 Neurotic 2 Analytically based 3 —	Clinical experience	Masochistic conditions if not too severe, impotence, organ neuroses.	Frigidity, considerable secondary gain, 'strong oral disposition'. Feasibility decreases with 'increasing depth of the neurotic disposition'.
Alexander (1944)	1 Neurotic 2 Analytically based 3 —	Clinical experience	Estimate of the 'functional efficiency of the ego' is of paramount importance.	

		Clinical experience	
Pumpian-Mindlin (1953)	1 Neurotic 2 Analytically based 3 —	Clinical experience	Patient has developed techniques of coping with situation so that he can get some satisfaction from human relations. Ability to tolerate frustration. Constructive interpersonal relationships. Ability to derive satisfaction from occupation and social activities. Disorder of recent origin.
Ripley, Wolf & Wolf (1948)	1 Psychosomatic 2 Eclectic, incl. supportive, expressive, abreactive, etc. Average 9 sessions. 3 889 patients. 1 year follow-up in 690.	'Symptomatic improvement: sustained diminution in symptoms and signs.' 'Basic improvement: meeting a major threat in life situation in a more constructive way and without symptoms.'	
Barron (1953a)	1 Neurotic out-patients 2 Interpretative, by residents. 3 33 patients.	Pre-treatment: MMPI. Outcome: Dichotomous scale, 'improved'—'unimproved', based on symptoms, personal relations, insight. 2 independent judges, close agreement.	Patients 'who are not very sick in the first place'. 'Unimproved' significantly higher on all MMPI scales. High on paranoia scale and those scales usually elevated in psychosis.
Barron (1953b)	Several different series.	Cross-validation of the 68 items on MMPI scale found most useful in previous study.	Good contact with reality, feeling of personal adequacy, lack of fear. He suggests that what is being measured by this scale is a general capacity for personality integration or ego strength.

Table 3—*continued*

Reference	1 *Type of patient* 2 *Type of therapy* 3 *No. of patients*	*Kind of evidence* *or criteria used*	*Good prognosis*	*Poor prognosis*
Rosenbaum, Friedlander & Kaplan (1956)	1 Neurotic out-patients. 2 Analytically based by trained but un-analysed residents. 9 months, once a week. 3 210 patients.	Statistical analysis of long questionnaire given to thera-pists. Outcome: 5-point scale, based on symptoms and social adjustment. Strict criteria. No statement of length of follow-up.	Ability to develop interpersonal relations. Good sexual adjust-ment. But no significant correl-ation with pre-treatment 'marital adjustment' or work adjustment.	
Sullivan, Miller & Smelser (1958)	1 Veterans, 25% psychotic. 2 Not stated. Median: 9 inter-views. 3 83 patients.	Pre-treatment: MMPI. Outcome: 'Improvement' on 5-point scale judged by therapists at termination.	'Improvers' have lower MMPI profiles than 'unimprovers', suggesting that 'improvers' are less sick in the first place.	

Probably the most widely held hypothesis about selection criteria is that *the prognosis is best in 'mild' illnesses of acute and recent onset.* For want of a better term I shall designate this throughout as 'Hypothesis A'.

This general criterion can be broken down into a number of separate but clearly interrelated criteria, as follows:

1. Mild psychopathology.
2. Sound basic personality, or high 'ego strength'—usually judged by the patient's ability
   (a) to cope with reality, and
   (b) to bear frustration and conflict.
3. History of satisfactory interpersonal relations.
4. Acute and recent onset of symptoms.

Opinions and work largely supporting these criteria are shown in *Table 3*.

The evidence in favour of Hypothesis A, therefore, might seem to be very strong. Nevertheless, there are to be found widespread through the literature strongly dissenting statements, clearly based on experience. Berliner (1941), for instance, rejects criterion 4 (recent onset), while retaining criterion 1 (mild psychopathology):

'In my experience this [referring to the statement by Knight (1937, see *Table 3*) in favour of Hypothesis A] is not quite so. In some of my cases the illnesses were of considerable duration and others were only acute reactions on the basis of a broader neurotic disposition. The feasibility of short treatment does not depend on the acuteness and duration of the illness but on the depth of the neurotic disposition.'

Pumpian-Mindlin (1953), on the other hand, falls even nearer to the 'radical' end of the scale, emphatically rejecting criterion 1, though retaining criteria 2 (ego strength) and 3 (satisfactory relations):

'First, I should like to point out an important negative finding for this type of therapy, namely, that short-term treatment is not dependent upon the amount or seeming severity of the psychopathology present in the patient nor upon the severity of the earlier traumata suffered by the patient. Our case material included cases of transvestitism, frigidity, colitis, pedophilia, depression, paranoia, impotence and various character disorders. The mere presence of severe psychopathology is no contra-indication to short-term therapy. Rather it appears to

depend upon other factors present in this group of patients—
which we might ordinarily sum up in the term "ego strength".'

Pumpian-Mindlin judges the relevant aspects of 'ego strength'
by the patient's ability to obtain satisfaction from personal
relationships, in spite of his symptoms, without being destructive
to himself or to others. He also mentions the ability to tolerate
frustration; and he makes a clear statement in favour of criterion
3, the 'adequacy of the patient's past and present object relationships'.

Similarly, at the first Brief Psychotherapy Council in Chicago
(1942; quoted by Gutheil, 1945), which was presided over by
Franz Alexander, good results were reported in psychopathic
personalities, character neuroses, delinquents, and psychotics.

Finally, the evidence provided by Stekel and his school is
equivocal. Many of their case histories—in which the therapeutic
result consisted of relief of single symptoms of recent origin—
clearly fit in with Hypothesis A. Gutheil (1933), who is one of
Stekel's pupils, writes: 'The shortest treatment is particularly
afforded in cases in which behind the neurotic symptoms an
actual conflict is hidden'—by which he means a conflict in the
patient's present life. At the same time Stekel's school—who expect
treatment to last for one to six months (Gutheil, 1933; Stekel,
1938)—recognize few limitations to their technique and take on
patients with psychopathology generally considered to be 'severe',
e.g. perversions, homosexuality, drug addiction, or psychosis.

Of course, without a full report and an adequate follow-up on
all these cases, the same objection can always be made as to the
results of the early analyses: namely, that the therapeutic results
consist of 'transference cures' or other kinds of 'false solution',
probably not lasting, and not in any way comparable with those of
long-term methods. Plenty of spokesmen for this aspect of the
'conservative' view can be found in the literature, mainly among
psycho-analysts. Thus, at the Brief Psychotherapy Council (quoted
by Gutheil, op. cit. 1945), N. C. Lewis was of the opinion that
'most of the briefer therapies yield only temporary results'; Rado
'considers brief psychotherapy as a technical procedure of a
palliative character . . . the aim is to relieve the patient from
certain symptoms that are painful or dangerous, or aid him in
handling a given situation or problem. Deeper changes in the
personality are neither attempted nor possible.'

Eissler (quoted by Murphy, 1958) says that:

'Psycho-analytic scrutiny will disclose that the majority of

22

cures by psychotherapy have been based on elaborate rationalizations which depend for their effectiveness on what is dynamically a repression of the basic conflict after some partial solutions of derivative conflicts have been attained and accepted as a compromise. In this sense psychotherapy has simply effected a change in the content of the neurosis or a re-channelization of libidinal energy based on displacement, or has led to new repression, or an exchange of illusions, the building up of magic beliefs or the development of an imitation of health.'

Eissler does, however, also express the following opinion, which is very important to any worker who is concerned with practical possibilities rather than perfection: 'Of course all such cures may be extremely worth while, lasting in effect and economically more feasible than results obtained in analysis.'

It is quite clear that one can multiply contradictory opinions of this kind indefinitely without being able to reach any conclusion. The only way of resolving the problem is to ignore opinions and to go direct to published case histories.

Unfortunately the problem here is exactly the same as with the early analyses. The amount of published work in which the therapeutic results are reported with sufficiently strict criteria, in sufficient detail, and with adequate follow-up, to survive inspection by the ruthless 'psychodynamic eye', is very limited. As has been pointed out by many authors, including Bandler (in Oberndorf, Greenacre, and Kubie, 1948) and myself (Malan, 1959), it is very necessary to exclude the possibility that a given improvement has been bought at the expense of a severe restriction in the patient's life. Bandler reported a gross example of this:

A girl when first seen suffered from agoraphobia, dressed very attractively, and complained about men's attentions. At follow-up she reported that there had been no recurrence of her agoraphobia, but now she dressed unbecomingly and complained that men weren't interested in her.

If the psycho-analytic view is adopted that agoraphobia is likely to represent sexual anxieties, then this girl obviously cannot be regarded as 'really' improved in spite of the fact that her symptom has completely disappeared.

Many of the published case histories do in fact fit in well with conservative views (i) of selection criteria, i.e. with Hypothesis A; and (ii) of results, in the sense that these consisted largely of symptom removal in otherwise apparently healthy personalities. Examples are shown in *Table 4*.

TABLE 4 CASE HISTORIES SUPPORTING CONSERVATIVE VIEWS

Reference	Patient Sex Age		Complaints	Duration of complaints	Type of treatment	Length of treatment	Outcome	Follow-up
Stekel (1923)	M	?	Patient was a priest complaining of an impediment in his speech affecting him in church services.	?	Stekelian analysis.	6/52	Symptom disappeared.	4 years
Knight (1937)	M	24	Frequent and imperative urination.	2 years	Analytically based interpretation, reassurance, advice.	3 sessions	Symptom disappeared.	6/12
Berliner (1941)	F	?	Obsessed with fear that she might cut the throat of her baby boy.	Presumably a few weeks	Discussion of ambivalent feelings, etc.	Few weeks	Great relief.	None
Alexander & French (1946)	M	51	Patient was a scientist. Severe revulsion against work. Extremely agitated. Couldn't speak without crying.	Few weeks	Analytically based interpretation.	2 sessions	Symptoms relieved. Few further mild depressions which did not seriously interfere with work.	8 years
Finesinger (1948)	F	30	Anxiety, nausea, vomiting.	?	Analytically based interpretation; support.	40 sessions	Marked improvement in symptoms.	None
Deutsch (1949)	M	28	Anxiety states, fugues, depersonalization, hypochondriacal ideas. Couldn't leave his mother.	2/12	'Associative' method with aim 'goal-limited adjustment'.	14	Symptoms improved but not cured. Left mother and married.	2 years (indirect)

There is, then, evidence at least for marked symptomatic relief in a number of cases; but cases other than those of Stekel and Alexander and French which were adequately followed up are very few indeed. Moreover, it has to be remembered that some of Stekel's case histories may possibly be fictitious (see Jones, 1955, p. 153). The documented evidence that brief psychotherapy is worth while even in those patients who fit in with Hypothesis A can thus hardly be described as satisfactory.

In fact, the evidence that patients with considerably more severe or more long-standing illnesses can also be helped is really little less satisfactory. The best documented of all the examples is probably that of 'Mrs. Oak', treated by client-centred therapy and reported in great detail with verbatim extracts by Rogers and Dymond (1954, see esp. pp. 262–3):

> The patient was a woman in her late thirties suffering from a deep disturbance in her personal relations, mainly with her husband and daughter. She also had never worked outside her home, and the prospect terrified her. The final therapeutic result was that (i) her relation with her daughter was much improved; (ii) she obtained a divorce by mutual consent and without too much bitterness; (iii) towards the end of therapy she 'chose an establishment in which she wished to work, applied for a position, ignored the turn-down which she received, and convinced the manager that he should give her a trial. She is still holding the position'; (iv) she felt that she was now ready to cope with life, though she knew it would not be easy; (v) she discovered a new ability to accept her femininity. (Forty sessions during $5\frac{1}{2}/12$; then a $7/12$ gap; then eight sessions during $2/12$; final follow-up $3/12$; follow-up since first termination nearly one year.)

The work of Thorne (1957) provides another indication of what may be achieved by intensive therapeutic effort and enthusiasm. Here the aim was to test eclectic psychotherapy on the most chronic and malignant cases that could still be treated as out-patients. Thorne emphasizes that the aim was reorganization of the personality in depth. Treatment averaged about forty sessions and seems to have been remarkably successful in a number of cases. Unfortunately the actual examples given are much longer than the above, so that none will be quoted here.

The only examples I have found of detailed accounts of relatively severe cases treated successfully, with a clear statement of long follow-up, are, once more, those of Alexander and French (op. cit. 1946). These authors report a number of cases of intermediate or moderate severity: e.g. a girl with a quite severe, though recent, generalized hysterical illness (Case K; twelve sessions; follow-up three years); a man with a five-year history of duodenal ulcer (Case L; thirty-seven sessions; follow-up two years); and a man of 24 who had suffered from attacks of bronchial asthma since the age of 14 (Case Q; *c.* forty sessions; follow-up three years). The most severe of all these cases is as below (Case O):

> The patient was a married woman of 50 who had suffered from gastro-intestinal distress and many other hysterical symptoms for twenty years, needing constant medical attention. Treatment consisted mainly of gradually uncovering the roots of her symptoms in self-imposed martyrdom in the home and rivalry with her daughter (fifty-eight sessions during one year). Follow-up (two years): only occasional gastro-intestinal symptoms.

The work of Alexander and French would suggest, therefore, that at least a few per cent of patients who do not fit in with Hypothesis A may yet be suitable for brief psychotherapy. This number is probably not too small for practical purposes, *provided such patients can be recognized with reasonable accuracy.* This brings us back once more to the problem of selection criteria— this time to those criteria which are relatively independent of the type or severity of the illness.

Now it is obvious that the ability to respond to brief psychotherapy must be a measure of some quality of *flexibility* in the patient, and the question arises whether such flexibility—or the corresponding contra-indication, rigidity—may not be recognizable independently in some way before therapy starts. This factor ('flexibility of personality structure') was regarded as of importance in the large-scale study by Ripley, Wolf, and Wolff (1948) where it was apparently assessed retrospectively by clinical judgement only. There is the great danger here of circular argument. A method of assessing the reverse of this factor, which is not open to the same objection, has however been discovered in an unexpected quarter, namely in a questionnaire test for *ethnocentrism*—which is a factor fairly certainly correlated with rigidity. A high score on this test was found by Tougas (in Rogers and Dymond, 1954) to be the best single way of retrospectively predicting outcome in client-centred therapy, and the same was found by Barron (1953a) for psychotherapy carried out by relatively untrained residents. This is an extremely interesting result, but it would perhaps be of less value in Britain where racial minorities are a less universal problem.

An important clinical way of assessing a factor connected with flexibility is emphasized by Alexander (1944), namely by making *trial interpretations*: 'The patient's reaction to such initial interpretations is the best guide in evaluating the patient's capacity for insight as well as the character and strength of his resistance and future cooperation.'

This criterion belongs to a group which we may call 'dynamic', as opposed to the more 'static' criteria concerned with psychopathology. Another member of this group is *high motivation* (mentioned by Ripley *et al.*, 1948; and by Knight, 1937, as probably correlated with acuteness). Correspondingly, Stekel (op. cit. 1938) seems to have regarded low motivation as almost the only contra-indication to his technique: 'Within a couple of months I can always discover whether the analysand's desire for illness exceeds his desire for help. . . . This willingness to be cured is of the utmost importance.'

These two last criteria will play an important part in the discussion of our own work.

Finally it might be expected that *projection tests* would be found useful; and particularly the Rorschach, which by now can be interpreted in such a highly reproducible way. Unfortunately there have been a number of studies which contradict this expectation. For instance, Barron (1953a) found that those patients who did and did not 'improve' (in psychotherapy with relatively untrained residents) did not differ significantly in any of the recognized scores or important ratios. Moreover, even experienced interpreters had little success in using the Rorschach protocols to predict outcome intuitively.

It will be seen that a study of the voluminous literature on this subject really leads only to a single conclusion: that *sometimes* striking therapeutic results can apparently be obtained in patients with relatively severe and long-standing illnesses. This does not necessarily contradict Hypothesis A, which can still be valid statistically. For the rest, it is scarcely possible to doubt that there is room for further investigation.

TECHNIQUE

Activity/Passivity

It is self-evident that a therapeutic technique which faithfully imitates that of analysis will inevitably lead in the end to nothing

27

other than analysis. Any technique of brief psychotherapy must therefore be based on differences from analysis, and particularly on a conscious opposition to one or more of the lengthening factors already described in Chapter 2. Of these, the most easily corrected is the analyst's tendency to passivity. The corresponding need for some kind of 'activity' in brief psychotherapy is one of the few matters of almost universal agreement in this whole field.

Passivity in analysis has many aspects: the use of the couch, of free association, the willingness to deal with whatever material the patient brings, the sense of timelessness. In most techniques of brief psychotherapy all these factors are corrected.

Several authors specifically mention that the couch should not be used (e.g. Fuerst, 1938; Stone, 1951) and probably most authors who do not mention this regard it as self-evident. The difference between the couch and the face-to-face technique is subtle but important. The two authors mentioned above emphasize that the use of the couch tends to lead the patient away from reality into phantasy, but this is not the only factor. The couch automatically encourages 'free association'—the tendency to describe into the empty air, so to speak, whatever passes through the patient's mind, with the corresponding tendency in the therapist to abandon initiative. The face-to-face technique creates an entirely different atmosphere in which the patient is talking not into the air but *to* the therapist. Therapy tends to become more of a dialogue, the therapist tends to take a more active part in the relationship, and the instruction to the patient to 'say whatever comes into his mind' seems rarely to be necessary.

The use of the face-to-face technique and the discouragement of free association are, however, only aids towards a more active handling of the patient's material. In Stekel's technique, for instance, this takes the form of active interpretation, particularly of the patient's dreams, based on free use of the therapist's previous experience and intuition. The great emphasis on dreams is clearly an attempt to by-pass the resistances and quickly enter the patient's unconscious world. It is interesting to note that, in contrast, several workers (e.g. Finesinger, 1948) discourage the interpretation of dreams for the same reason as they discourage free association, because they feel it leads away from reality.

A different aspect of 'activity' is emphasized by several modern schools of brief psychotherapy, and forms one of the principles on which there is the greatest measure of agreement. This comprises several related principles: that the therapist must first of all abandon another of the lengthening factors, namely therapeutic perfectionism, and *plan* a *limited aim* from the beginning, pursuing it by *guiding* the patient by means of some technique of *selective attention*. The terms used by Finesinger (1948) are 'goal-directed planning and management' and the 'focusing of material'; those used by Deutsch (1949) are 'goal-limited adjustment' and 'sector therapy'. The particular method of selective attention used by Deutsch is called by him the 'associative anamnesis'—which consists of repeating and emphasizing significant words or phrases used by the patient, and thus inducing further associations in a direction which the therapist has selected. Similarly Pumpian-Mindlin (1953) says that the patient may be guided by 'skilful neglect'.

Pumpian-Mindlin makes a specific statement concerned with abandoning therapeutic perfectionism:

'Both patient and therapist must be able to accept improvement or "cure" in terms of the presenting problems and feel reasonably satisfied with this. The therapist must not feel forced to work for any deep-going character transformation. . . .'

In Alexander and French (op. cit. 1946) there is a chapter written by French entitled 'Planning psychotherapy', in which many of these interrelated themes are touched on in the following passage:

'. . . the temptation is very great merely to treat the patient's problems as he brings them to us and thus, as it were, to let the patient drift into an analysis. . . . It is highly important, therefore, to outline as soon as possible a comprehensive therapeutic plan, to attempt to visualize in advance (even if only tentatively) just what we shall attempt with our patient, what we hope to accomplish. . . .

In order to do this, it is necessary, first, of course, to make a dynamic formulation of the patient's problem. . . . After outlining all the possibilities and rejecting those that may be dangerous or impractical, he [the therapist] will outline his plans for helping the patient to achieve those that seem to be realizable.'

Little further comment is needed, except to emphasize once more the substantial and unusual measure of agreement among different authors.

After all this emphasis on the necessity for activity, planning, and selective attention, it seems strange to turn to a school of brief psychotherapy whose basis is a technique *more passive than*

29

that of analysis, namely client-centred therapy (see Rogers, 1951). Here the therapist refuses to make inferences of any kind (which are of course the basis of interpretations), and confines himself to the 'reflective' technique, simply clarifying the essential feelings which the patient has already expressed openly. Ideally, two things happen which also happen in analysis, but to a greater extent than in analysis: (i) the patient experiences the therapist as someone who accepts him, identifies with him, values him, and makes no other judgements at all; and (ii) the patient achieves insight—but not from the therapist—on the contrary, entirely through self-examination. That far-reaching changes can be achieved in certain cases by means of this technique has already been discussed (p. 25).

How 'deep' to go

The vague word 'deep' is used deliberately here, since it covers a number of different aspects of technique which are conveniently discussed together. The word has the following connotations: (a) far from consciousness, (b) disturbing, and (c) belonging to an 'early' stage of development. Since one of the lengthening factors is the therapist's preoccupation with ever 'deeper' and 'earlier' feelings, it is clear that one way of shortening therapy may be to keep interpretations more 'superficial'. Whether or not this is sufficient to give the patient worth while help is a matter for experience to decide.

This leads to a very important question of technique: whether the therapist (a) should make his interpretations only in terms of the *current* life problem, the relation to people in the patient's *present* life, or *external* reality; or (b) should not be afraid where necessary to make interpretations about the roots of the patient's neurosis in *childhood,* his relation with his *parents,* or his *inner world.*

On these questions there is some of the widest divergence of all between the conservative and radical views. Examples of quotations lying at the conservative end of the scale are:

> Fuerst (1938): 'The technical aim is not so much to make unconscious material conscious as to build up an Ego, which can handle the conflicts of the present situation. Generally we are not able to deal with material which belongs to deeply repressed unconscious layers (oral and anal material).'

> Finesinger (1948): 'When used in relatively brief psycho-therapy, it [i.e. insight therapy] seldom exposes the phantasies

and memories that are most deeply repressed. . . . Dream or phantasy material is seldom used for interpretation excepting when a more extensive therapy is undertaken.'

Pumpian-Mindlin (1953): 'Interpretations . . . are couched in more general terms and not related to necessarily specific historical conflicts and difficulties in the patient. In addition, the interpretations are usually made not in terms of unconscious underlying impulses but in terms of the more readily available preconscious material. One works primarily with the reverberations of earlier conflicts as they are reflected in adult and adolescent behaviour and attitudes rather than attempting to uncover the genetic childhood conflicts *per se.*'

The more fearless radical view is not often stated explicitly, but is quite clearly implied by Stekel and by Alexander and French. The implications of these workers' case histories are that no limits can be set beforehand; that the therapist should go as 'deep' as is necessary to help the patient; and that sometimes, for instance, a conflict should be interpreted in terms of the present only, and sometimes it should be traced to its roots in childhood. (As an example of the former, see Alexander and French, Case B: a scientist of 51 whose problem was interpreted only in terms of competition with his younger colleagues; of the latter, see Case P: a young man of 19 whose severe depression was resolved by uncovering his feelings about his mother's death when he was 3.) Alexander makes clear in many of his writings (e.g. Alexander, 1944) that he regards 'psychoanalytic therapy' and gull-scale analysis as forming a continuum.

This leads to a third and most important question of technique, namely the use of transference. Here there is an exactly similar divergence of views.

Transference
It should be noted first of all that the word 'transference' can be used in three different ways: (a) to denote any feelings that the patient may have for the therapist, (b) to denote only those feelings that are neurotically based, and (c) to denote only those feelings specifically derived from infantile life. The second meaning will be adopted throughout the present work.

As has been discussed in Chapter 2, one of the characteristics of the 'primitive' technique of the early analysts was the absence of transference interpretations; and perhaps the most important of all the lengthening factors has been the development of, and the necessity for resolving, the transference neurosis. One of the fundamental questions of brief psychotherapy is therefore whether the transference neurosis can be avoided.

There is universal agreement that it should and can be avoided, but this is where the agreement ends. Obviously the development of any kind of transference must carry the danger of the ultimate development of a transference neurosis. The question is then whether any transference should or can be avoided or discouraged, should be ignored if it develops, should be diverted, should be interpreted only when absolutely necessary, should be interpreted without fear, or should even be encouraged. A complete spectrum of views from the most conservative to the most radical occurs.

The conservative view is carried to the limit by the client-centred therapists, who state that with their technique transference can be largely avoided, and that the factor responsible for this is not merely the absence of transference interpretation, but the absence of interpretation of any kind. The following quotations are from Rogers (1951):

'The possibility of effective brief psychotherapy seems to hinge on the possibility of therapy without the transference relationship, since the resolution of the transference situation seems to be uniformly slow and time-consuming.'

'With many clients the attitudes toward the counselor are mild, and of a reality, rather than a transference, nature. . . . If one's definition of transference includes all affect towards others, then this is transference; if the definition being used is the transfer of infantile attitudes to a present relationship in which they are inappropriate, then very little if any transference is present.'

'In psycho-analysis these attitudes develop into a *relationship* which is central to the therapy. . . . In Client-centred Therapy, however, this involved and persistent dependent transference relationship does not tend to develop. Thousands of clients have been dealt with by counselors with whom the writer has had personal contact. In only a small minority of cases . . . has the client developed a relationship which could in any way be matched to Freud's terms.'

Rogers suggests that as soon as the therapist makes an interpretation he inevitably implies that he knows better than the patient, and often implies a value judgement; and that this leads to a crumbling of self-confidence in the patient and to a dependent relationship with the therapist. This explanation strikes me as superficial, but I have no better one to offer. Whatever the true explanation, the apparent absence of transference in client-centred therapy demonstrates clearly the profound influence of technique on the kind of response produced in the patient.

Of course the technique of reflection is only of theoretical interest to psycho-analysts, who are irrevocably committed to the use of interpretation. Of these, Deutsch seems to represent the most conservative in attitude to transference. In his book (Deutsch, 1949), which gives a complete account of one therapy, I have found no transference interpretations at all. Another conservative author is Pumpian-Mindlin (1953), with whom the emphasis is both on avoiding and on diverting the transference:

'In short-term therapy there is a general tendency to avoid an intense transference and to take measures to diminish the transference phenomena which inevitably appear. Mechanically this is accomplished by means of less frequent visits and by implicitly or explicitly structuring therapy in terms of the circumscribed presenting problem only.'

'An interesting technical device with regard to the use of transference . . . consisted of deflecting the specific problems being dealt with in therapy onto an important figure in the patient's environment rather than focussing the problem around the patient-therapist relationship.'

Certain authors lying towards the centre believe that it is sometimes necessary to interpret the transference, but only when it begins to disturb the therapy, particularly when it becomes used as resistance or becomes 'negative'. These views imply that the transference is a necessary evil, and thus can be compared with the views of psycho-analysts in the middle period:

Berliner (op. cit. 1941): 'There must be a good positive transference during the whole period so that no time has to be spent on transference analysis. Of course transference analysis is done immediately when it is indicated (that is when resistance arises from it). But it needs more time and the treatment may take the course of a full analysis. The amount and power of the transference resistances is a decisive factor in the question of the feasibility of short treatment. The analyst has to do his share in keeping the transference positive.'

Stekel (op. cit. 1938): 'But whereas no allusion should be made to the positive transference unless it interferes with the analysis, immediate steps must be taken to obviate a negative transference. Hate must be diverted onto its primal cause.'

The radical end of the scale is best represented by Alexander and French. In their flexible approach, transference interpretation may play any part. They quote cases in which transference interpretations were not used at all; cases in which some aspects of transference were handled by interpretation and others by acceptance; and finally cases in which the main aim of the whole therapy was to give the patient a new kind of experience in his relation with the therapist. This last is what these authors call the 'corrective emotional experience':

'reexperiencing the old, unsettled conflict *but with a new ending* is the secret of every penetrating therapeutic result. Only the actual experience of a new solution in the transference situation or in his everyday life gives the patient the conviction that a new solution is *possible* and induces him to give up the old neurotic patterns.'

Here the primitive, conservative view of transference—even the negative transference—as a necessary evil has entirely disappeared. This view is indistinguishable from the most modern view of the therapeutic action of psycho-analysis.

LENGTH OF TREATMENT, TERMINATION, AND FOLLOW-UP

So far no attempt has been made to define any arbitrary point at which therapy ceases to be 'brief' and becomes 'long-term'. Obviously the definition of brief psychotherapy must depend on experience of what gives satisfactory results. A study of those 'successful' cases of which some details have been actually published allows only the following generalizations to be made:

1. Quite far-reaching changes can be obtained in certain cases in 10–50 sessions (Alexander and French; Rogers and Dymond).
2. (a) Case histories of 1–4 sessions are to be found fairly widely in the literature: Alexander and French, five cases; Saul (1951), one case; Rothenberg (1955), three cases; Knight (1937), three cases; Berliner (1941), one case.
   (b) It may possibly be true that it is these cases that tend to fit in with Hypothesis A. Of the above cases only those of Saul and of Berliner possibly fail to fit in with this idea.

Termination and follow-up are very little discussed in the literature and, although these questions will be shown to have

34

played a very large part in our own work, they can be dismissed briefly here. Only Stekel (op. cit. 1938) seems to discuss the problem of resentment at termination. Most of the other passages where termination is mentioned imply that termination should be considered either when there is danger of drifting into long-term therapy (Pumpian-Mindlin, op. cit. 1953), or when there has been sufficient therapeutic gain (Alexander and French, op. cit. 1946, pp. 36–7). The device of setting a time limit from the very beginning was adopted by Seitz (1953) in the treatment of 'psychocutaneous excoriation syndromes'—a very honest account of an experiment which was therapeutically not an unqualified success. Phillips and Johnston (1954) applied this idea to child-guidance interviews, feeling that it was important for therapy to have a definite beginning, a middle, and an end. They found, in sixteen cases treated with this device, a higher proportion of 'improvement' and of 'mutually agreed termination', and a lower proportion of 'premature withdrawal', than in fourteen cases treated conventionally.

The problem of leaving the patient-therapist relationship in such a state that the patient is willing to return for follow-up also does not seem to be discussed, though there are some indications in the literature that this is indeed a problem. Thus Seitz (1953), in the experiment described above, was able to contact only five out of twelve 'improved' patients one year after termination; and two of these, who had relapsed, 'politely declined' when offered further treatment. Similarly, the patient described at length by Deutsch (1949) managed to avoid follow-up altogether, though Deutsch obtained information about him through his father.

PREVIOUS WORK: CONCLUSION

The foregoing review will have amply demonstrated the present state of confusion in this field. Of the few tentative conclusions that can be drawn, the most important is that there is considerable evidence against the conservative view of brief psychotherapy, at least in individual cases; but, on the other hand, whether such cases represent an appreciable proportion of the population, and how they may be recognized, is almost impossible to tell.

The major deficiencies in the literature lie in the following:

1. The failure to publish sufficient details of individual cases, with the result that an independent observer is rarely able to draw his own conclusions;

35

2. The tendency to select only the most successful cases for publication, so that no lessons are learnt from failures;
3. The utter neglect of the vital necessity for developing psychodynamic methods, based on published evidence, for assessing therapeutic results;
4. The partial neglect of the equal necessity for long follow-up.

The reader should be left in no doubt that a study that satisfied no more than the three criteria below would meet a pressing need:

1. All cases treated were published in some detail;
2. Results were assessed psychodynamically on published evidence;
3. Strict attention was paid to follow-up.

The present study was undertaken with this need in mind.

PART II

THE PRESENT WORK

CHAPTER 4

Preliminary

DESCRIPTION OF PATIENTS, THERAPISTS, AND METHODS OF WORKING

Patients

The study to be described here is based on a total of twenty-one therapies, representing all those cases—with one exception— formally taken on by the team and either *definitely terminated* or *definitely abandoned to long-term therapy* between January 1955 (when the whole project started) and the end of January 1958. The one exception (the Transvestist) is a patient who was in fact formally taken on, but who was quite clearly unsuitable for psychotherapy of any kind, with whom the therapist could make no contact whatsoever, and who finally drifted away from therapy without apparent improvement after a total of about five sessions. This patient made so little impact on the members of the team that he was simply ignored or forgotten—he was never included in our interim reports and no attempt was made to follow him up. This is a scientific oversight for which I can only apologize. By January 1958, also, another patient (the Car Lady) was clearly expected to end up in long-term treatment (she had so far had twenty-two sessions and the prospect of termination seemed remote); but although this expectation was subsequently fulfilled, she has not been included. It has been necessary to draw a firm line somewhere, or the work would have been never-ending.

The patients were all taken from those referred routinely, or with a special request for immediate help, to the Tavistock Clinic in London (eighteen patients) or the Cassel Hospital in Richmond (three patients).

Members of the Research Team

The team will often be referred to by its nickname, 'the Workshop', from now on. The Workshop consisted of members of the staff

39

of the Tavistock Clinic and the Cassel Hospital (with the exception of Mrs. Balint, who has been closely associated with the work of the clinic for many years).

The composition of the Workshop varied. The maximum strength (excluding visitors) was nine. In the twenty-one cases considered, there were seven different therapists. It is necessary to state that all the therapists must be regarded as skilled: by the time that they entered this work, all had had several years' experience of psycho-analysis and/or analytically based psychotherapy. Only one had not yet started his training as a psycho-analyst; the rest were either recently qualified as analysts or became so during the course of the work. All cases were under the constant supervision of the whole team, led by Dr. Balint, who can claim to be one of the most experienced analysts—both in clinical work and in teaching and supervision—in Britain today.

Method of Working

The Workshop met once a week for $1\frac{1}{2}$–2 hours for discussion of current cases. Abbreviated transcripts of these discussions, taken down in shorthand at the time, were circulated and preserved. Accounts of the therapeutic sessions were dictated by the therapists from memory.

As already noted, emphasis was more on clinical enthusiasm than scientific discipline. Although, therefore, attempts were made to state hypotheses, therapeutic plans, and predictions in a formal manner, in the heat of the discussion these attempts were often unsuccessful. No attempts were made at any time to score judgements for statistical purposes. Judgements often, and scores always, have to be inferred retrospectively from the case records and the transcripts of the discussions, with all the scientific dangers that this entails. Judgements, when made, were by consensus of opinion—in Balint's words, 'knocking our heads together until something comes out of it'—which has its own advantages, like trial by jury.

Nevertheless, strictness of *clinical* discipline leaves little to be desired. All patients but one (the Paranoid Engineer, a psychotic patient for whom it was thought at the time to be inappropriate) were given a projection test before, or early in, therapy. This was either the Rorschach or the 'Object Relations Test' ('ORT': Phillipson, 1955), a psycho-analytically based form of the TAT. Both tests were interpreted intuitively, along psycho-analytic lines, by experienced psychologists (Mr. Boreham, Mr. Phillipson, or Mr. Rayner—usually Mr. Boreham). There was full discussion

of all patients either before they were taken on or early in thera
Sessions were reported to the Workshop verbally at freque
intervals, and were thoroughly discussed. During these discussions
therapists were frequently cross-examined, and were not allowed
to get away with very much in the way of distortion or suppression
of evidence.

COURSE OF THE WORK

The work opened with a long preliminary discussion of our
preconceptions about brief psychotherapy, based mainly on casual
first-hand experience. From this a single clear trend can be seen
in retrospect to have emerged: that the views expressed were
overwhelmingly conservative. For selection criteria, we all
favoured Hypothesis A. For technique, we were mainly preoccupied with fear of the transference neurosis; and consequently
our discussions were much concerned with ways in which the
transference could be avoided, deflected, or ignored. It is important
to note, therefore, that our original intention amounted to an
attempt to 'turn back the clock' and return to the primitive technique of the early analysts.

The immediate aim then became that of a pilot study: to select
patients thought to be suitable, to apply the techniques suggested,
and to see what therapeutic results could be achieved. That this
plan reckoned without the powerful ecological factors at work in
the interaction between a population of patients and a group of
well-trained psycho-analysts will be discussed in later chapters.
Suffice it to say that neither as far as selection criteria nor as far
as technique were concerned were we able to hold to the original
intentions. We tended to choose the patients in whom we were
interested; and we used the technique which came naturally to us.
The result was, by chance, a great gain both in the scientific and in
the therapeutic value of our work. Having begun by being highly
conservative, we ended as radical as almost any previous worker in
this field.

SCOPE OF THE PRESENT STUDY

The rest of this book will consist of a detailed presentation and
discussion of the evidence provided by these twenty-one therapies
on the questions of :

1. Therapeutic results
2. Selection criteria
3. Technique.

The present work

The greatest emphasis of all will be laid on the presentation and assessment of the results. This is not only the major unsolved problem in the whole field of psychotherapy; but it must necessarily form the central part of any study of this kind, upon which almost all other conclusions depend.

There are perhaps one or two dozen important and interesting topics that have not been explored at all, of which a few are: (i) the relation between therapeutic plans and actual events; (ii) the relation between the evidence provided by the psychiatric interview and the projective test; (iii) what follow-up means to the patient. There are also fascinating clinical points illustrated by many individual patients. I have confined myself almost entirely to an overall view of the work and to principles that are of general application.

CHAPTER 5

The Assessment of Therapeutic Results

This very difficult problem was the subject of a separate paper (Malan, 1959). The whole difficulty may be illustrated by a single example, the agoraphobic girl quoted by Bandler (in Oberndorf, Greenacre, and Kubie, op. cit. 1948) and already mentioned in Chapter 3 (p. 23). The essential point illustrated by this patient is that (i) while she dressed and behaved in such a way that men were attracted by her, she suffered from agoraphobia; and that (ii) when she lost her agoraphobia, she was found to have changed her behaviour in such a way that men were no longer interested in her. It is thus hardly difficult to postulate (i) that the agoraphobia and the problem of her relation to men were dynamically linked, (ii) that the 'real' underlying disturbance lay in her relation to men, and (iii) that there had therefore been no *resolution* of her 'real' problem, which on the contrary had been solved merely by *avoidance*. In other words, emotional health cannot simply be equated with the absence of symptoms. It is hardly necessary to drive this home by drawing the medical parallel, and discussing whether freedom from pulmonary tuberculosis should be equated with the absence of cough.

Adherents of the psychodynamic view have of course recognized this distinction between 'symptomatic' and 'real' improvement for many years. Various terms have been used for the latter: 'basic' improvement (Ripley, Wolf, and Wolff, 1948); 'specific' improvement (Kessel and Hyman, 1933); 'improvement in the pathological condition' (Alexander, 1937); and of course many authors speak of 'character changes'.

This is the problem—how to recognize 'basic' or 'specific' improvement; what is meant by 'character changes'; how to tell that there has been improvement in the 'pathological condition'; or, in terms adopted in my previous paper, how to distinguish between 'resolution' and various kinds of 'false solution', of which 'flight into health' and 'transference cure' are the most familiar examples.

The medical analogy may be pressed further in illustration. The first step in considering a patient is to draw up a list of *symptoms and signs*. The next step, making a *diagnosis*, consists in formulating an *explanatory hypothesis* linking the symptoms and signs together as manifestations of known *pathological processes*. Here the principle of economy of hypothesis is brought into action, that is, the minimum number of pathological processes is postulated—if possible, of course, only one.

In medicine the nature of most pathological processes is very fully understood. It is therefore possible to lay down an exact theoretical meaning of true 'resolution' of the illness—in pulmonary tuberculosis, the death of all tubercle bacilli and the cessation of the inflammatory reaction. This cannot usually be directly observed, but theoretical and empirical knowledge can be used to provide *criteria of presumed resolution* which are more reliable than the mere absence of symptoms: e.g. information from the sputum, the sedimentation rate, or x-rays; and the large body of empirical knowledge about the course of the illness, which makes possible the assumption that if all known manifestations have not recurred within a certain time it is safe to return the patient to a normal life.

Now although in psychodynamics the difficulties are much greater, the principles used can be exactly the same. First of all, it is possible to draw up a list of the known disturbances in a patient's life. The search for these can be greatly assisted— exactly as in medicine—by empirical and theoretical knowledge: if a patient complains of night sweats, it is natural for a physician to inquire about cough and loss of weight; if a patient complains of agoraphobia, it is natural for a psychiatrist to inquire about sexual inhibition. Moreover, whether or not the psychiatrist believes that the sexual inhibition and the agoraphobia are psychopathologically connected, the sexual inhibition—if found— is *there* and must be taken into account in any assessment of the patient's emotional health.

But here the parallel with medicine begins to break down. The diagnosis of 'agoraphobia', in contrast to that of 'pulmonary tuberculosis', implies nothing that is nearly so generally accepted about an underlying pathology; nor, as with 'progressive muscular atrophy', for example, does it even imply an illness of insufficiently understood pathology, the future course of which can be predicted with reasonable certainty.

Nevertheless, these difficulties can be partly overcome. First, since an independent observer must be enabled to judge any evidence for himself, the list of disturbances must be set down in full. Next, psychodynamic theory is used to formulate a hypothesis by means of which these disturbances may be linked together. Since, to a far greater extent than in physiological illness, no single patient is like another, each particular patient requires a separate hypothesis. The principle of economy of hypothesis is here used in two ways: (i) as in medicine, the minimum *number* of hypotheses; and (ii) as in any science, the minimum *amount* of theory is used by means of which the disturbances may be linked. This whole process is best illustrated by a simplified example from our own work:

The patient (the Articled Accountant), a young man of 22, was sent for treatment after an acute outburst of uncontrollable homosexual feelings. Interview revealed the following:

1. that the homosexual feelings appeared soon after a girl in the office had shown some interest in him (the patient said, 'homosexual feelings seemed easier somehow');
2. that he had hardly been aware before this of sexual feelings directed towards either sex;
3. that he had an obsessional fear of making small mistakes at work, was afraid of his boss, and was afraid particularly that his boss would find out about his relation with the girl.

Now these facts may, if the reader chooses, be regarded as unrelated. At the same time, if a hypothesis can be found that plausibly fits them all together, it must deserve consideration. The following hypothesis fulfils this:

This patient's 'main problem' is an intense fear that male authority figures will disapprove of his heterosexual feelings, which has caused him to retreat into homosexuality.

It should be noted that the absolute minimum of psycho-dynamic theory has been used. Nothing, for instance, is said about the original cause of this patient's fear—though a hypothesis is of course ready to hand in the psycho-analytic theory of the Oedipus complex. Although more might well be needed for therapy, nothing more is needed for an assessment of the therapeutic result.

Now, in the present state of our knowledge, it is not possible to lay down criteria by which the underlying pathological process can really be judged to have been 'resolved'. For this reason, the words 'resolved' and 'resolution' are used mainly for their brevity and are not intended to imply any firm theoretical basis. It is possible, however, to state criteria by which it can be judged that *all known manifestations of the original disturbance have disappeared.* This, quite clearly, means the disappearance not only of the 'positive' neurotic manifestations but of the inhibitions and restrictions as well; that is, not only that homosexual feelings should be greatly reduced in intensity, but that heterosexual feelings should appear in their place; not only that direct fear of the boss and obsessional anxiety about mistakes should disappear, but that the patient should become confident in his work, and that he should establish a satisfactory relation with his boss based neither on excessive submissiveness nor on excessive hostility.

The principles used here can be generalized and illustrated in the following way: first, a basic tenet is that evidence taken from changes in the patient's phantasies, or in his behaviour with the therapist, or in his reaction to projection tests—though of course it may be very important—is not accepted unless it is supported by information about changes in the patient's life *away from the clinical situation.* (This does not necessarily mean externally observable changes or changes in behaviour—changes in feeling, for example a reduction in anxiety, are of course accepted also.) In the next example this condition was not fulfilled:

> Another young man (the Civil Servant) gave, in his projection test immediately after therapy, clear evidence that he had been deeply affected by his relation with the therapist. Now the therapist was a woman, and one of his main disturbances was an inability to make contact with women. Yet, at follow-up three years later, his relation with girls was still almost entirely in the imagination; and this disturbance must necessarily be regarded as 'essentially unchanged'.

Second, a 'disturbance' in a patient's life means some kind of reaction which is judged to be neurotic or *inappropriate*; and in the best possible therapeutic result this 'inappropriate reaction' must not merely have receded or disappeared, but must have been *replaced* by the corresponding 'appropriate reaction'. Moreover, where the inappropriate reaction is to a symbolic situation, for example the Articled Accountant's obsessional anxiety about mistakes, the corresponding appropriate reaction is a reaction to a situation in which the *symbols have been translated* (here, guilt about mistakes at work is taken to represent guilt in relation to male authority about heterosexuality, so that the appropriate reaction will have to be sought in his relation to both of these). The exact interpretation of neurotic symptoms such as obsessional or phobic anxieties, or of psychosomatic symptoms such as headache, is never easy to guess before therapy has provided the evidence needed, and is often not easy then. Here the principle has been adopted of basing the psychodynamic hypothesis—if possible—mainly on the more direct evidence from the disturbances in human relations, and of assuming that each symptom is some kind of expression, symbolic or psycho-physiological, of the conflict involved—often a symbolic compromise between the unconscious impulses seeking expression and the repressing forces. There is no need to be more exact, because the assessment criteria automatically require that the symptoms and the disturbances in human relations shall both be substantially reduced.

Nevertheless, the majority of patients show only partial changes, and the result may then be much more difficult to assess. The principles adopted here are as follows:

1. *Partial resolution*
(a) Substantial improvement in the human relations without improvement in, but without exacerbation of, the symptom.
(b) Limited improvement in both the human relations and the symptom.

2. *Clear-cut false solution*
Loss of symptom, with solution of the problem of human relations by withdrawing from it.

The third case is much more difficult:

3. Loss of symptom, with minimal changes in the problem of human relations.

This requires illustration and discussion:

The example is once more the Civil Servant. The disturbances in this patient included (a) agoraphobia, (b) an inability to make contact with girls, and (c) obsessional anxiety about small mistakes, with great anger if criticized by male authority. The psychodynamic hypothesis is, once more, fear of being punished for heterosexuality by male authority figures, with corresponding anger against them. The agoraphobia is assumed to represent some kind of sexual anxiety. The result of therapy consisted of complete disappearance of the agoraphobia with minimal changes in the other disturbances. How should this result be assessed?

47

I am far from denying the value of removing a symptom such as this—which was making the patient's life a misery before therapy—as long as the improvement is not bought (as it was in Bandler's case quoted on p. 23) at the price of a new severe restriction in the patient's life. This kind of result is therefore regarded as 'worse' than one in which there was definite evidence for 'partial resolution', but 'better' than 'essentially unchanged'.

There is another kind of result which I regard as having a similar status. This is what I call the 'valuable false solution'—in which, although the changes that occur show no evidence for genuine resolution, they unquestionably reduce the strain in the patient's life at a price judged to be not too heavy—for instance by causing a benign circle to be set up, or a vicious circle to be prevented. If, for example, an impotent man is enabled to restore his defences and recover his potency, immense harm may be prevented from being done to his relation with his wife. Similarly, even the temporary 'transference cure' is not to be underestimated, if it results in a decision by the patient (for instance to make a reasonably happy marriage, see the Surgeon's Daughter) which has lasting beneficial effects on the future.

There are obvious difficulties here. One is that for the necessary information one has to rely entirely on the patient, who may of course distort the facts for many reasons and in many different ways. This objection is not as serious as it may seem. In the first place, a dynamically conducted interview with interpretation is the most effective way of exposing such a distortion—and it is a virtue of almost all psycho-analysts that they are utterly ruthless in the scrutiny not only of other people's therapeutic results, but also of their own (see, for an example of this, the follow-up of the Draper's Assistant). In the second place, any method of assessment in which the patient is aware of the significance of the information that he supplies, including such apparently 'objective' methods as the 'self-ideal correlation' of Rogers and Dymond, is open to exactly the same objection—even more so, as there is in these methods no way of exposing distortions such as there is in a psychiatric interview.

There are yet other problems more especially concerned with the present work. At what point is 'brief' therapy regarded as a failure because it has now become 'long-term'? The policy is adopted here of defining 'brief' therapy in terms of the length envisaged in the original plan or decided during therapy, allowing a good deal of latitude for difficulties over termination or the later continuation of a loose therapeutic relation. Thus, for the

Hypertensive Housewife, 'brief' therapy is taken to have ended at the first attempt at termination, after nineteen sessions, and the continuation of regular sessions (20–39) is regarded as 'long-term'; while, on the other hand, the forty sessions of the Falling Social Worker, who was set a time limit of three months at three times a week from the beginning, are all regarded as 'brief'.

This leads to the question of patients who have undergone and have maintained partial improvements, but are much later taken on for long-term therapy because they or the therapist hoped for more. Is the mere fact of their being taken on again to be regarded as indicating that the original brief therapy was a failure? I have adopted the opposite point of view: that provided a reasonable time has elapsed since the original termination, the original improvements should be allowed to stand—otherwise the status of the result depends on factors quite independent of the changes themselves, such as whether the patient asks for further treatment or not, or whether there is a vacancy for him. The result is that further follow-up uncomplicated by the new course of therapy becomes impossible, but this has to be accepted.

Finally, a difficulty which runs throughout this whole discussion is that phrases such as 'inappropriate reaction', 'satisfactory relation', or 'valuable false solution' not only leave much to be desired in exactness and objectivity, but also imply judgements of value, and may even mean 'taking sides' in the patient's struggle with his environment. For instance, it may well be judged that a healthy reaction for a daughter would be to leave a possessive mother, but what about the point of view of the mother? I believe that this difficulty is unavoidable and has to be faced; and that this can be done by stating the values openly and making the judgements on published evidence, so that an independent observer is free to disagree with them. The values used are mainly those derived from psycho-analysis: that, on the whole, human beings are happier if they are always free to use either their basic instinctual drives, or the forces restraining these, in a given situation; and that there usually exists an *optimum* and *relatively high level* at which these drives can be used, above *and* below which not only the individual suffers but also his environment. The criterion that can often be used is thus the effect on both: for example, it is assumed that both the Articled Accountant and his boss would find their relation more satisfactory if the former became less afraid and more self-assertive. The actual result, however, in which the patient had a series of rows with his boss and finally gave in his notice without foreseeing the problem of references, is regarded merely as the replacement of one inappropriate reaction by another.

There are further values which must also be stated. These are: (i) that, on the whole, relations with *people* are regarded as more important than relations with *things*; (ii) that, also on the whole, relations with marriage partners or people of marriageable age of the opposite sex are regarded as more important than any other relations; and (iii) that great importance is attached to heterosexual satisfaction. These values become of importance in 'three-person' problems such as that of the Articled Accountant —for instance, an improvement in his relation with male authority would be regarded as less important than one in his relation with girls.

In the present series of patients I have not found these hypotheses and judgements very difficult, for they really consist of no more than a formalization of the Workshop's consensus of opinion. This is, however, unquestionably partly due to the special characteristics of these highly selected patients, to the high level of emotional interaction between patients and therapists at the original interviews—which resulted in very clear psychodynamic material—and to the almost unrivalled experience in psychodynamic diagnosis of Balint himself. It must be emphasized also that, since *these patients were used retrospectively for developing this method of assessment*, there is much hindsight in both judgements and hypotheses, and that the whole method thus appears much easier than it would be if carried out entirely prospectively. Nevertheless, I do not believe that it would be impossible.

For statistical purposes these results are scored on a four-point scale ('resolution' is used as shorthand for 'replacement of inappropriate by appropriate reaction'):

Score 3: Evidence for substantial resolution in the main problem.

Score 2: Evidence for limited resolution in the main problem— particularly resolution in the problem of relations with the same sex without change in relations with the opposite sex.

Score 1: (a) Substantial symptomatic improvement without appreciable changes in the problems of human relations.
(b) Valuable false solution.

Score 0: All other changes or no change.

50

CHAPTER 6

Assessment and Therapy Forms

NOTES ON THE ASSESSMENT AND THERAPY FORMS

As has already been discussed, I hold the opinion that an essential factor in any research in psychotherapy is the publication of a summary of the evidence on all the patients treated. This evidence is set down in 'Assessment and Therapy Forms', one of many such forms developed by the Workshop for the purpose of summarizing clinical material. It has been necessary to strike a balance between completeness and unmanageable length. For this reason I have concentrated mainly on what I regard as really essential: (i) a full account of the original disturbances in the patient and the changes in them, and (ii) a brief account of the course of therapy. I have in general omitted the material provided by projection tests and interviews by independent assessors, except where this provides important additional or contradictory information. There is no intention of underestimating the contribution of our psychologists, which in almost every case formed an integral part of the initial assessment, and in several an integral part of the assessment of the therapeutic result.

I regard the great length of this section as unavoidable. Almost the whole of the rest of the work depends on the evidence presented here. The reader will wish to be selective, and I would suggest some of the following as representative of both satisfactory and unsatisfactory results and assessments:

1. The Biologist and/or the Neurasthenic's Husband: examples of striking and clear-cut results in relatively severe illnesses.
2. The Girl with the Dreams: a fair result, with an unsatisfactory and highly intuitive assessment.
3. The Unsuccessful Accountant: a clear example of what is meant by 'valuable false solution'.
4. The Storm Lady: an example of a dramatic therapy which ended in failure to terminate.
5. The Student Thief: a presumed failure with an assessment rendered very unsatisfactory by failure of follow-up.

TABLE 5 INDEX TO PATIENTS AND ASSESSMENT AND THERAPY FORMS

Patient	Sex	Age	Complaint (duration)	Diagnosis	Therapist	Total sessions	Duration of therapy	Score for outcome	Page
Articled Accountant	M	22	Homosexual feelings of acute onset (8 weeks).	Homosexuality; reactive depression.	F	27	13 months	0	56
Biologist	M	27	Eating phobia (3½ years).	Phobic anxiety; latent homosexuality.	B	10	5 weeks	3	61
Civil Servant	M	22	Agoraphobia and eating phobia (6 months).	Phobic anxiety.	A	12	6 months	1	66
Clown	M	24	Lack of self-confidence, feeling that people look at him (13 years).	Character disorder; reactive depression.	B	5	4 weeks	–	70
Dog Lady	F	33	Severe phobia of dogs (27 years)	Phobic anxiety.	F	10	5 months	–	74
Draper's Assistant	F	21	Non-consummation of marriage (7 months).	Frigidity; phobic anxiety.	A	10	5 months	0	77
Falling Social Worker	F	27	Phobia of falling (10 years).	Phobic anxiety.	G	40	4 months	3	80

Girl with the Dreams	F	24	Disturbing dreams (several years), recent acute panic attack (2 months)	Anxiety-hysteria.	A	18	8 months	2	84
Hypertensive Housewife	F	34	Depression (4 years).	Severe reactive depression.	D	19	6 months	0	89
Lighterman	M	30	Anxiety attacks of acute onset (2–3 months).	Compulsive neurosis; post-traumatic syndrome.	F	17	15 months	3	93
Neurasthenic's Husband	M	50+	Complex character difficulties including inability to deal with his wife (over 15 years).	Character disorder.	E	14	5 months	3	99
Paranoid Engineer	M	28	Fear that he may be homosexual (at least 5 years).	Borderline paranoid psychosis.	F	13[a]	8 months	0	104
Pilot's Wife	F	24	Frigidity (10 months).	Hysterical personality.	F	19	12 months	0	107
Railway Solicitor	M	24	Headaches (2½ years).	Anxiety neurosis; reactive depression.	G	30	3 months	3	111

Table 5—continued

Patient	Sex	Age	Complaint (duration)	Diagnosis	Therapist	Total sessions	Duration of therapy	Score for outcome	Page
Storm Lady	F	23	Severe phobia of death and storms (about 20 years).	Phobic anxiety state; underlying depression.	B	19[a]	6 months	0	115
Student Thief	F	20	Stealing (2 weeks; possibly 1–2 years).	Pathological stealing.	F	11	4 months	0	119
Student's Wife	F	27	Phobia of falling (11 months).	Phobic anxiety.	G	9	2½ months	0	123
Surgeon's Daughter	F	29	Unmarried pregnancy (6 weeks).	Character disorder; reactive depression.	C	18	10 weeks	1	127
Tom	M	16	Anxiety attacks of acute onset with physical symptoms (4 weeks).	Severe anxiety-hysteria.	B	4	4 weeks	0	132
Unsuccessful Accountant	M	31	Inability to get a job (2 years).	Character disorder.	F	7	6 weeks	1	136
Violet's Mother	F	42	Acute family crisis (5 weeks).	Neurotic marital problem.	F	15	5 months	0	140

[a]Failure to terminate.

6. The Student's Wife: a clear-cut failure.

7. The Clown: a complex result, probably a failure, which has been found impossible to assess.

Certain notes are required:

1. The summaries of therapy have been made by myself, and do not necessarily correspond with summaries that would have been made by the actual therapist (where this was not myself). These summaries are, however, based not only on the written case notes, but also on the 'living' accounts of most sessions given by the therapist at the meetings.

2. It has not always been possible to give the response to interpretations because this would often mean the inclusion of excessive detail. I hope enough examples appear to give an impression of what is meant by a 'marked' response—a concept that is unmistakable but almost impossible to define.

3. The forms are arranged in alphabetical order of pseudonyms. An index (*Table 5*) is included on pp. 52–4.

4. A summary of the therapeutic results, arranged according to the type of problem treated, is shown in *Table 6* (pp. 142–8) at the end of the forms.

5. Throughout the whole of the rest of this study the names of members of the staff who had contact with the patients are suppressed; otherwise patients might be more easily identified. The number of children in the patient's family and the patient's position among siblings have been omitted for the same reason. The relation between a patient and his siblings played very little part in these therapies. The case histories are mostly somewhat disguised. Those of the Lighterman and Articled Accountant were published in a more heavily disguised form in my paper (1959).

6. Two cases only, the Falling Social Worker and the Railway Solicitor, were treated as in-patients. Sessions were mostly once or twice a week. All patients were treated face to face.[1]

7. (a) Sessions are numbered from the first interview (not counting the projection test) with a Workshop member. The initial interview therefore is often the same as 'session 1'.

   (b) 'Length of therapy' is measured from session 1 to final termination.

   (c) 'Length of follow-up' is measured from date of termination.

[1] Except the Dog Lady who was treated on the couch for one or two sessions and who then asked to sit with her back to the therapist.

THE ARTICLED ACCOUNTANT

A. DETAILS OF PATIENT AND THERAPIST

1. *Patient*

Sex   M
Age   22
Marital status   Single
Occupation   Articled to a chartered accountant.
Complaint   ⎫ Acute appearance of uncontrollable homo-
What seems to bring   ⎬   sexual feelings, leading to homosexual
  patient now   ⎭   behaviour in public, for which he was
                            arrested.

2. *Therapist*

Code   F
Sex   M

B. PSYCHIATRIC HISTORY AND DIAGNOSIS

Family history. NAD

Home atmosphere. Happy

Previous history. NAD

Diagnosis. Homosexuality and reactive depression in an obsessional and inhibited personality.

C. ALL KNOWN DISTURBANCES IN PATIENT'S LIFE

(a) *Homosexual feelings*
These appeared suddenly after a girl in the office had shown some interest in him. He got himself picked up by another young man. The relief which he sought was obtained when the other man touched his (the patient's) genitals.

(b) *Inhibited heterosexuality*
Largely unaware of heterosexual feelings. Masturbates without phantasy; has nocturnal emissions without dreams. Has never tried to have a girl friend though he has mixed freely with both sexes at school and at college.

(c) *Depression*
After appearing in court he was afraid he would not be allowed to continue as an accountant and he could not face his parents. He experienced a terrible sense of depression and intended to go home, not tell his parents, and commit suicide with an overdose of aspirin. He was saved by the fact that his parents had already been told

what had happened by his boss. He was treated for depression by his GP and was no longer depressed when seen by us.

(d) *Relations with older men*
Unable to stand up to his boss and another older man in the office; feels uneasy with them; constantly worried about making small mistakes. Always feels uneasy at doing something which his father wouldn't do.

(e) *Denial of experience*
Does not know what he wants out of life. Never planned his career, just drifted into it. Avoids unpleasant feelings by denying them or filling his life with something else.

D. AREAS OF PATIENT'S LIFE UNAFFECTED BY ABOVE DISTURBANCES
Fair academic history, about in keeping with his potentialities. Good, very close, non-sexual relations with young men of his own age.

E. MINIMUM PSYCHODYNAMIC HYPOTHESIS SUGGESTED TO EXPLAIN C
Fear of being punished for heterosexuality by a male authority, with flight into homosexuality. His defence against conflict of all kinds is a denial of feeling.

F. EVIDENCE REQUIRED IN ASSESSMENT OF 'IDEAL' RESULT
(a) No further homosexual feelings.
(b) Active attempts at forming relations with girls, with ultimate success.
(c) No further serious depression.
(d) Satisfactory relations with older men based neither on excessive submissiveness nor on hostility; ability to stand up to them; no uneasiness in relation to them; no further worry about small mistakes; able to do things without guilt that his father wouldn't do.
(e) Ability to experience feelings freely, especially unpleasant feelings. Clear knowledge of what he wants out of life, with active planning for the future.

G. THERAPEUTIC PLAN FORMULATED AT INITIAL ASSESSMENT
To interpret the Oedipal problems leading to a flight from heterosexuality.

H. SUMMARY OF COURSE OF THERAPY
Although this pleasant and sincere young man rarely responded dramatically to interpretations, he obviously understood them and

57

The present work

(*The articled accountant—continued*)
worked with them steadily. In sessions 1–11 the therapist concentrated on interpreting the homosexual episode as expressing (i) *a flight from heterosexuality* (the girl in the office) and (ii) *the need for love and affection from his father* (who had become much more distant when he returned from the war). Steady progress was made and the patient's confidence at work markedly increased.

During this period evidence that the patient wanted a longer relationship with the therapist became apparent in session 4, and was interpreted without very much effect in sessions 4–7.

The clearest material came in session 12, with a dream in which the patient had in his possession a key that he had no right to. The therapist interpreted that this represented *his father's penis, which the patient felt he had to steal in order to become a man*; and that when he and the young man had touched each other's genitals he was seeking reassurance that they did not want to castrate each other. There was no dramatic response to this interpretation, but in session 13 the patient came up full of confidence, and the therapist suggested *beginning to tail off treatment*. In session 14 the patient, in a state which—seen in retrospect—was probably somewhat hypomanic, had a long phantasy about the sweeping changes he would make in the office if his boss retired.

WORK ON TERMINATION. In session 15 the patient was not nearly so cheerful, and in session 16 he reported that he had been *depressed*. Depression steadily deepened during subsequent sessions. *Anger and a sense of loss at termination, related to the failure of the relation with the patient's father*, were made into a focus during sessions 15–22. Finally, in session 22, there was a clear response to the interpretation that the patient wanted things to go wrong at work so that he could say it was his boss's fault. The therapist suggested that the patient had felt the same about therapy, with the implication that this partly accounted for the relapse and depression, but this the patient denied. In the next session, however, he reported a *sudden lifting of his depression*.

> Total no. of sessions 27
> Total time 13 months

I. CHANGES IN ALL DISTURBANCES LISTED UNDER C

Follow-up (1) 2 months:

(*a*) *Homosexual feelings.* Now has no wish to seek a homosexual relationship actively, but has homosexual feelings at times, and 'I don't know what I'd do if someone tried to seduce me'.

(*b*) *Heterosexual feelings.* One half-hearted attempt during therapy to form a relationship with a girl was revealed as an attempt to please the therapist, and came to nothing. He is still unaware of heterosexual feelings; still masturbates without phantasy; still has nocturnal emissions without dreams. His close male friends have moved away and he is solitary, spending his week-ends alone.

(*c*) *Depression.* None.

(*d*) *Relations with older men and work.* Has considerably improved in his ability to stand up to his boss and another man in the office —if anything he has gone the other way, and treats his boss with lack of consideration. Great increase in his confidence and ability to enjoy his work. No further worry over small mistakes. His ability to enjoy things his father wouldn't do has increased.

(*e*) *Denial of experience.* Little permanent change. Has tentative plans about leaving home and changing his job, but gives the impression he is waiting for something to turn up.

Follow-up (2) 7 months:

(*a*), (*b*), and (*c*). No further change.

(*d*) and (*e*) *Relations with older men and work; Denial of experience.* After the recent death of his father, which he experienced quite deeply, he has been determined to get what he can out of life before it is too late, and has also been having rows with everyone, including his boss.

Follow-up (3) 2 years 7 months:

(*a*) and (*b*) *Sexual problems.* No further change.

(*c*) *Depression.* He said that he had had a number of attacks of mild depression, each lasting for a short time only, since the last follow-up; but that the last was a considerable time ago.

(*d*) *Relations with older men and work.* His relation with his former boss ended in a serious row and the patient gave in his notice. This made references very difficult, but the patient has now got a job as managing clerk in an accountant's office. He gets on well in the direct relation with his present boss, in spite of the fact that the boss tends to be rude. Nevertheless, he is over-anxious about making mistakes when he is given responsibility; and at one point, when he nearly got the firm into trouble, felt he would have to give up accountancy altogether, even though his boss was not much worried about it.

The present work

(*The articled accountant—continued*)

(*e*) *Denial of experience.* He has given up all idea of taking his final exams and becoming a chartered accountant, though he knows he could perfectly well do so if he chose. He is solitary and lonely, most of his friends having moved away, and he doesn't know how to set about making new ones. His feelings about his father and the therapist now seem very far away. He is, however, still able to enjoy things his father wouldn't have done.

J. PSYCHODYNAMIC ASSESSMENT OF RESULT

The main inappropriate reaction (homosexuality) has *receded* without being replaced by the corresponding appropriate reaction (heterosexuality).

Secondary inappropriate reactions:

1. *Fear of male authority.* At first replaced by another inappropriate reaction—excessive hostility. Possibly now replaced by appropriate reaction, but evidence from his relation with his present boss is not sufficient.
2. *Obsessional anxiety about mistakes.* Possibly somewhat reduced but clearly still present.
3. *Depression.* The tendency towards depression seems to be still present.
4. *Denial of experience.* After initial replacement by appropriate reaction this has re-formed, and is now unchanged.

Summary. Insufficient evidence of improvement for an assessment higher than 'essentially unchanged'.

Score 0.

K. STATUS OF THE EVIDENCE

The psychodynamic evidence is unequivocal, and there seems little justification for a score higher than 0.

This patient is very similar to the Civil Servant, who also shows a recession of the inappropriate reaction without replacement by the appropriate reaction. The essential difference between the two seems to be as follows: the present patient has given up all attempts at forming relations with girls, and has quite unnecessarily abandoned attempts to realize his full potential at work. The Civil Servant, though he has had little success in either field, is still trying in both. This is why the Civil Servant scores 1 and the present patient only 0.

THE BIOLOGIST

A. DETAILS OF PATIENT AND THERAPIST

1. *Patient*

Sex	M
Age	27
Marital status	Married
Occupation	By training a biologist, but now doing administrative work for a firm dealing in pest control.
Complaint	Difficulty over eating in public (3½ years).
What seems to bring patient now	Has only five weeks in London in which to get help.

2. *Therapist*

Code	B
Sex	M

B. PSYCHIATRIC HISTORY AND DIAGNOSIS

Family history. NAD

Home atmosphere. 'Happy and united.'

Present illness. Sudden onset 3½ years ago. Symptoms somewhat variable but essentially the same since then. GP treated him with alkalies at first, and two years ago he had an appendicectomy, without relief in either case. Patient states that Ba meal was negative.

Mental state. Patient gave a somewhat paranoid account of relations at work.

Diagnosis. Phobic anxiety, conversion hysteria, and latent homosexuality in a possibly paranoid personality.

C. ALL KNOWN DISTURBANCES IN PATIENT'S LIFE

(a) *Eating phobia*
This arises only when he eats in public and not at all at home. The worst kind of occasion is a business meal. He works himself up three or four days beforehand; during the actual morning he becomes tense, cannot keep still, trembles and sweats, but is conscious of little overt anxiety. He begins to feel sick but has never actually vomited. His 'stomach muscles bunch up' and he

61

(The biologist—continued)

has pain below the ribs. During the meal itself the food seems to get stuck below his ribs. He is afraid that he will vomit in public and that he will get left behind and become conspicuous. All this is greatly relieved at the end of the main dish. He always has indigestion afterwards.

(b) *Sexual difficulties*

(i) *Heterosexuality.* Poor erection and premature ejaculation ever since marriage (two years). Getting bored with married life.

(ii) *Homosexuality.* Has recently found homosexual impulses, which were strong at school, returning. He has attacks of compulsive phantasies with a clear homosexual flavour.

(c) and (d) *Difficulties with older men and achievement*

His eating difficulty manifests itself particularly in the presence of his superior at work. Follow-up revealed difficulties over work (see below).

D. AREAS OF PATIENT'S LIFE UNAFFECTED BY ABOVE DISTURBANCES

He presents a very good front and has so far done very well at work.

E. MINIMUM PSYCHODYNAMIC HYPOTHESIS SUGGESTED TO EXPLAIN C

Guilt and anxiety about repressed homosexual impulses, now returning to consciousness. Therapy suggested that these impulses, at least partly, represented submissiveness covering anxiety about competition with men.

F. EVIDENCE REQUIRED IN ASSESSMENT OF 'IDEAL' RESULT

(a) Disappearance of eating phobia.

(b) (i) Disappearance of potency difficulties, with improvement in enjoyment of sexual intercourse. Improvement in his relation with his wife.

    (ii) Disappearance of homosexual impulses and phantasies.

(c) and (d) Improvement in relations with men. No problems over work or achievement.

G. THERAPEUTIC PLAN FORMULATED AT INITIAL ASSESSMENT

The following plan was formulated after the initial interview:

1. To see him twice a week for the time available (five weeks).
2. To find out and interpret the meaning of the eating phobia.

(The biologist—continued)

After session 1 it was suggested that the therapist should concentrate on passive homosexuality.

H. SUMMARY OF COURSE OF THERAPY

This patient, who gave the impression of a well-educated, successful business executive, was first seen by a non-Workshop member, and then for an ORT by his therapist. During both these interviews he denied that his symptom had a psychological origin. Some interpretative work was done in the ORT, and in session 1 the patient's first recorded remark was that he now felt that his problems were psychological. He then at once plunged into unconscious communication, talking mainly about his relation with older men, while the therapist concentrated on interpreting rivalry and aggressive feelings. When this session was reported in the Workshop, the suggestion was made that *passive homosexual feelings* would have been more appropriate, and this became the main focus for the rest of therapy. In session 3 the patient was in resistance, and this was resolved by the first transference interpretation—the need to keep the relation with the (male) therapist under control. The patient responded by saying that he knew he was going to have to talk about his home life but had been consciously trying to avoid it. This led in session 4 to the patient's talking about his father, with interpretations about his attempt to deny that he felt more of a man than his father. In session 6 the interpretation was made that his *fear of vomiting represented his fear of showing the guilty shameful things inside him*—perhaps something to do with masturbation. The patient responded by telling of an incident at school in which he had been *caught masturbating with another boy* and a prefect had made hints about this at a *meal table*. In session 8 a number of interpretations were made about the patient's wish for a passive homosexual relation with the therapist. The session threatened to develop into an argument and interpretations about negative transference brought out a small amount of hostility. In session 9 the patient reported that he had *been to the firm's annual luncheon*—usually the worst occasion of the year for him—*almost without anxiety*.

WORK ON TERMINATION. In session 10 several interpretations about the patient's uneasiness over termination were made, with some agreement from the patient but no marked response.

Total no. of sessions 10

Total time 5 weeks

The present work

I. CHANGES IN ALL DISTURBANCES LISTED UNDER C

At termination:

(*a*) *Eating phobia.* Had been to the firm's annual luncheon with hardly any anxiety at all.

(*b*) *Sexual difficulties.* (i) *Heterosexuality*: Potency considerably improved but 'not 100 per cent'; (ii) *Homosexuality*: Homosexual phantasies 'completely gone'.

(*c*) and (*d*) *Difficulties with older men and achievement.* Apart from the disappearance of the eating phobia, which manifested itself particularly in the presence of his superior, no information. Now, however, preoccupied with a need to be '100 per cent virile'.

Follow-up (1) 8 months:

No further change except emergence of a new problem:

(*d*) *Difficulties over achievement.* Not working as well as he used to. Getting unhappy at work. 'People standing in the way of his promotion.' Thinking of changing his job.

Follow-up (2) 3 years:

(*a*) *Eating phobia.* No recurrence.

(*b*) *Sexual difficulties.* (i) *Heterosexuality*: Improvement in potency maintained. Now 'a happy united family'; (ii) *Homosexuality*: The homosexual phantasies had been largely absent, though with a few minor recurrences, until the demotion at work (see below). They then returned in full force. He got so desperate that he 'went down on his knees and prayed for help'. The phantasies disappeared and have been absent since then (1 month).

(*d*) *Difficulties over achievement.* He left his previous job and got a managerial position at another firm. He began to get behind in his work and was demoted. Now looking for other jobs, without success so far, and feeling desperate.

Follow-up (3) 5 years:

(*a*) *Eating phobia.* No recurrence. The only manifestation now is that he gets a feeling of fullness after eating only a little, but this does not worry him.

(*b*) *Sexual difficulties.* (i) *Heterosexuality*: Whole family very much happier. 'Contented domestic scene' in the evenings. No premature ejaculation, can wait until wife is ready. Intercourse mostly at week-ends, but nearly always entirely satisfactory to both partners.

(ii) *Homosexuality*: The homosexual phantasies have returned to some extent; he now gives in to them 'about once a month'. The recurrence occurred at about the time he got the present satisfactory job (see below).

(*c*) and (*d*) *Difficulties with older men and achievement.* Two years ago he got a job as second in command in a small firm. He is very happy in this job, and is earning and doing well.

J. SUMMARY OF CHANGES. PSYCHODYNAMIC ASSESSMENT OF RESULT

(a) Almost complete and permanent disappearance of symbolic representation of problem (eating phobia).
(b) Fluctuations, and ultimate reduction, in homosexual tendencies—though not complete disappearance by any means. Marked improvement in relation with opposite sex, including sexually. Almost certainly 'sublimation' of some of the homosexuality in his relation with his new boss (regarded as a satisfactory solution).
(c) and (d) Problem of competition and achievement apparently satisfactorily solved, though partially by avoidance. 'Valuable false solution' to this particular problem.

Complex, but score 3.

K. STATUS OF THE EVIDENCE

The psychodynamic evidence is extremely clear. According to the evidence it would be difficult to score this result any lower.

THE CIVIL SERVANT

A. DETAILS OF PATIENT AND THERAPIST

1. *Patient*

Sex	M
Age	22
Marital status	Single
Occupation	Junior civil servant.
Complaint	Agoraphobia and fear of eating in public, six months.
What seems to bring patient now	The anxiety developed shortly after he was given the job of answering inquiries by the public in his office.

2. *Therapist*

Code	A
Sex	F

B. PSYCHIATRIC HISTORY AND DIAGNOSIS

Family history. NAD

Home atmosphere. Undisturbed, though there was probably lack of contact between the patient and his parents.

Previous history. NAD

Present illness. Sudden onset; symptoms have continued ever since.

Diagnosis. Phobic anxiety-hysteria in an obsessional, immature, and inhibited personality.

C. ALL KNOWN DISTURBANCES IN PATIENT'S LIFE

1. Known at initial assessment:

(a) *Psychosomatic and anxiety symptoms*
(i) Permanent feeling of faint sickness.
(ii) Feeling of sickness greatly increased, and in addition there appear dizziness and sweating of palms, if in a situation from which he cannot escape without attracting attention—evening classes, theatre (cinema is all right), waiting for a coach with a party of people. Usually manages to stick this out, e.g. the second hour of evening classes is not too bad.

(iii) Sickness and anxiety symptoms greatly increased also if he has to eat in public, e.g. in a restaurant, but can force himself to do so. Recently lost his appetite when some people came to dinner at home.

(b) *Difficulty with girls*

Cannot make contact with girls. Has never taken a girl out. Had to give up attempt to learn to dance. Cannot show girls in the office how to do their jobs.

(c) *Obsessional phenomena—Difficulty with authority—Anger*

Constantly worried about making mistakes, and particularly about discussing them with his father. Gets very angry and feels he would like to kill anyone who tells him off about making a mistake— particularly the head of his department at work, who is very unpopular with everyone.

2. Which came to light during therapy:

(d) *Problems over achievement and competition*

These at the moment seem to be fairly mild. His academic career seems not quite up to his potentialities. Much preoccupied with his achievement in sport, at which he does quite well.

D. AREAS OF PATIENT'S LIFE UNAFFECTED BY ABOVE DISTURBANCES

Is doing tolerably well at work, enjoys his recreations, and is struggling hard to manage in spite of his phobias.

E. MINIMUM PSYCHODYNAMIC HYPOTHESIS SUGGESTED TO EXPLAIN C

Guilt and anxiety about sexual feelings towards women, much of which is based on a strong, guilt-laden feeling of rivalry and hostility towards men. His phobias are assumed to be a symbolic representation of aspects of this conflict, but their exact meaning is not clear.

F. EVIDENCE REQUIRED IN ASSESSMENT OF 'IDEAL' RESULT

(a) Complete relief of his anxiety.
(b) Active attempts to make relationships with girls, without undue anxiety, and with ultimate success. Ultimately, full potency.
(c) Improvement in his relation with male authority, based neither on excessive hostility nor on submissiveness. Ability to stand being criticized.

(The civil servant—continued)

G. THERAPEUTIC PLAN FORMULATED AT INITIAL ASSESSMENT

To interpret, as forcefully as possible, anxieties derived from the Oedipus complex.

H. SUMMARY OF COURSE OF THERAPY

This young man was described by the therapist as looking frightened, underfed, and unloved. He treated the therapist very 'nicely' and she felt it important to get at the negative feelings behind this façade. The transference focus of inability to contradict the therapist was interpreted without much response in sessions 3, 4, 5, 7, and 8. This was related to the patient's anger with his father and fear of getting into conflict with him. In session 7 the patient had quite a *heated disagreement with the therapist*, and this open expression of feeling (which the therapist pointed out) represented perhaps the moment of greatest communication in the therapy. In subsequent sessions the atmosphere changed. There seemed to be a secret, anxiety-laden, pleasurable relationship with the therapist as a woman, which the patient was not able to admit openly in spite of the therapist's attempt to bring it to the surface. A number of non-transference interpretations were made about sexual anxieties. The patient worked with them but never responded markedly. He finally felt he would like to manage on his own, and the therapist agreed.

WORK ON TERMINATION. None recorded.

Total no. of sessions   12
Total time   6 months

I. CHANGES IN ALL DISTURBANCES LISTED UNDER C

Latest follow-up: 2 years 11 months (interview with independent assessor).
Previous follow-up interviews: 3 months; 1 year 9 months; 2 years 6 months.

(*a*) *Psychosomatic and anxiety symptoms.* The agoraphobia, eating phobia, and feeling of sickness completely disappeared soon after termination, and have not returned. He has gone to evening classes without trouble. He sometimes has anxiety at office dinners, but sometimes enjoys them. Otherwise no trouble.

About one year after termination, however, he began to suffer from a lumpy feeling in his throat, which is present most of the time but does not worry him much. He feels this represents the anger he doesn't allow to come out. This is the first time he has openly accepted a psychological explanation for any of his symptoms.

(*b*) *Difficulty with girls.* His relation with girls remains largely idealized and in phantasy. He is strongly affected by girls he sees in the train. He has taken girls out on about two occasions, but they didn't come up to his expectations and he dropped them. He feels he couldn't take a girl home to his parents.

(*c*) *Obsessional phenomena—Difficulty with authority—Anger.* He is worried that his parents will find out about small mistakes, less worried that his boss will do so. At work, however, he does have to check things more than most people, and this makes him slow.

As far as anger is concerned, the information is equivocal. He told the therapist (2 years 6 months) that he probably gets angry more easily than most people, but verbalizes his anger and this only seems to lead to good results. He told the independent assessor (2 years 11 months)—with whom he was clearly angry at the time—that he often got angry with people, didn't show it, and a long time later might have an imaginary conversation in which he said all the things he would like to have said.

(*d*) *Problems over achievement and competition.* He has now failed his final exams twice, but is going on trying.

J. SUMMARY OF CHANGES. PSYCHODYNAMIC ASSESSMENT OF RESULT

Disappearance of phobic symptoms, with emergence of a now much milder psychosomatic symptom. Probably no essential change in problems with girls, men, anger, or competition: i.e. marked recession of symbolic inappropriate reaction without replacement by appropriate reaction.

Score 1.

K. STATUS OF THE EVIDENCE

Information full: interpretation fairly certain.

THE CLOWN

A. DETAILS OF PATIENT AND THERAPIST

1. *Patient*

Sex	M
Age	24
Marital status	Married
Occupation	Laboratory assistant.
Complaint	Self-consciousness, lack of confidence; feeling that people look at him; thirteen years.
What seems to bring patient now	Probably the fact that his first baby was born a few weeks ago, but patient is not conscious of this.

2. *Therapist*

Code	B
Sex	M

B. PSYCHIATRIC HISTORY AND DIAGNOSIS

Family history. Father suffers from peptic ulcer. Mother, very nervous, cries a lot.

Home atmosphere. Constant family quarrels as long as he can remember.

Previous history. Enuretic till 14. Married eighteen months.

Diagnosis. Long-standing character disorder with a paranoid element, now with reactive depression accompanied by anxiety.

C. ALL KNOWN DISTURBANCES IN PATIENT'S LIFE

(a) *General problems*
Feels people look at him. Now finding it increasingly difficult to work because of this. He left a previous job because people made mild fun of him—felt angry, couldn't express it, unable to talk to them, left. When embarrassed his brains 'seem to jam like a calculating machine' and he feels his face becomes frozen and people can 'label him'. Unable to take responsibility. Defends himself against all these feelings by deliberately playing the clown.

(b) *Depressive manifestations*
Feels no use. Future seems empty. Has crying attacks.

(c) *Problems connected with masculinity*

After initial difficulties the sexual relation with his wife is fairly satisfactory. He feels it is slightly distasteful to ejaculate inside her. He can satisfy her but is somewhat disappointed himself. He cannot realize he is now a father. He is especially self-conscious in the presence of virile men.

(d) *Problems over work*

He is thoroughly dissatisfied with his present work and wants to work in the country.

(e) *Manifest anxiety*

Between initial interview and projection test he got into a state of severe anxiety.

D. AREAS OF PATIENT'S LIFE UNAFFECTED BY ABOVE DISTURBANCES

He managed to go through with marriage against his father-in-law's wishes. The quality of the relation with his wife is fair—he says it depends on his dominating her and taking the decisions.

E. MINIMUM PSYCHODYNAMIC HYPOTHESIS SUGGESTED TO EXPLAIN C

1. Severe anxieties about attaining masculinity, exacerbated by recently becoming a father. The depression is probably reactive to his feeling of failure as a man.
2. There also seem to be much deeper disturbances of a paranoid kind.

F. EVIDENCE REQUIRED IN ASSESSMENT OF 'IDEAL' RESULT

(a) and (b) Extensive reduction in feelings listed under (a) and (b) above, with increase in self-confidence and ability to get on with people.
(c) Full satisfaction from sexual intercourse; evidence of his ability to take his place as father in the home, and to cope in competition with men.
(d) Solves his problem over a job realistically and gets satisfaction from it.
(e) Disappearance of state of severe anxiety.

G. THERAPEUTIC PLAN FORMULATED AT INITIAL ASSESSMENT

To concentrate on interpreting anxieties about fatherhood and to try to avoid dependent transference.

The present work

(The clown—continued)

H. SUMMARY OF COURSE OF THERAPY

The patient was in a state of severe anxiety after the initial interview, demanding immediate help or he couldn't carry on. The therapist consistently tried to apply the plan of interpreting problems concerning masculinity, but the patient always came back to demanding advice about changing his job. In session 4, after very little apparent progress, he said he was already looking for a job in the country. Nevertheless he said he had got what he wanted from the therapist—he had been made to feel a human being, not a flop or a fraud. At the last moment the therapist, feeling that neither he nor the patient was really satisfied, asked if there was something more that the patient wanted to discuss. The patient immediately said that there was something he very much wanted to ask: 'Whether you think that there is anything about my face that would make people look at me.' The therapist suggested that he needed to appear as a clown because he was afraid of appearing as a man, and then he felt people looked at him. The patient seemed very content with this interpretation, and parting was on a note of great warmth. He was seen once more, briefly. He had got a job as a farm labourer many miles from London and seemed very happy.

WORK ON TERMINATION. The only hint of this was the therapist's question, in session 4, whether the patient was satisfied with the work done, to which the answer was affirmative (see above).

Total no. of sessions   5
Total time   4 weeks

I. CHANGES IN ALL DISTURBANCES LISTED UNDER C

Follow-up (1) 1 year 9 months:

The follow-up interview revealed a very complex situation:

(a) General problems. He says he now has no social anxieties—he can joke with people and carry on normal conversation—but he says that this is *entirely dependent on his taking drugs* prescribed for him by his GP. If he stops taking drugs he says his voice goes husky, and he feels himself going down and down and he retires into his shell. This would probably make him unable to go to work. In contrast to the original feeling that his thoughts get frozen if he feels people are making cutting remarks, his mind tends to race. He says he has given up playing the clown, but he feels he might become a bore and people would think him silly.

Towards the end of the interview, he gave what seemed to be a

(*The clown—continued*)

quite paranoid account of his first experience of being tested at the clinic.

(*b*) *Depressive manifestations.* No certain information, presumably much improved.

(*c*) *Problems over masculinity.* He now has two children and feels he is a success as a father. He is very happy with his wife and says the sexual relation is very good. He feels that this change is not dependent on his taking drugs. He has a feeling of achievement in being able to support his family.

(*d*) *Problems over work.* He stayed in the farm job only for a few weeks, and since then has had three jobs, all below his capacity, the last for two months. He seems content nevertheless.

(*e*) *Anxiety.* Completely disappeared.

Follow-up (2) 2 years 10 months:

Letter from psychiatrist saying patient had been referred to him and asking for a report. Therapist wrote and asked for information about patient's present condition, but received no reply.

J. SUMMARY OF CHANGES

At follow-up (1) both his social difficulties and those over masculinity seem to have been largely replaced by the appropriate reaction; but much of this improvement—possibly all—is dependent on taking drugs. The work problem remains. The anxiety has disappeared. Follow-up (2) gives us no more information than that he has sought treatment again.

Result probably essentially unchanged, but really impossible to assess.

No score.

K. STATUS OF THE EVIDENCE

Very incomplete.

THE DOG LADY

A. DETAILS OF PATIENT AND THERAPIST

1. *Patient*

Sex	F
Age	33
Marital status	Married
Occupation	Housewife
Complaint	Intense fear of dogs since the age of 6.
What seems to bring patient now	Afraid that her daughter, now aged 2, will become affected by this fear.

2. *Therapist*

Code	F
Sex	M

B. PSYCHIATRIC HISTORY AND DIAGNOSIS

Family history. Father has been diagnosed as anxiety neurosis.

Home atmosphere. Father used to have violent rages. Mother nagged father and 'finally won domination over him'. Constant quarrelling between parents in front of children. One brother very withdrawn, could not settle in any job.

Present illness. Phobia has hardly fluctuated in intensity since it began.

Diagnosis. Phobic anxiety neurosis.

C. ALL KNOWN DISTURBANCES IN PATIENT'S LIFE

1. Known at initial assessment:

(a) *Dog phobia*
'Absolutely terrified' of dogs. Cannot pass a dog in the street—has to cross to the other side or run into the nearest garden. Much more afraid if the dog barks. Leaves the house only when absolutely necessary, two to three times a week.

(b) *Need to control people*
Some evidence at interview, abundantly confirmed later, that she arranges things so that everybody is nice and kind to her, and finds it difficult to tolerate if people don't fit in with this.

2. Which came to light during therapy:

(c) Need to run away from treatment repeatedly and be persuaded back. She failed to come to the first appointment offered but came

(*The dog lady—continued*)

to the second. This pattern was manifested frequently during the whole period of short- and long-term therapy.

(d) Terror of having group treatment.

D. AREAS OF PATIENT'S LIFE UNAFFECTED BY ABOVE DISTURBANCES

She has functioned well in all the externals of life at the price of her severe phobia.

E. MINIMUM PSYCHODYNAMIC HYPOTHESIS REQUIRED TO EXPLAIN C

The evidence suggests that she is very afraid of some kind of primitive feeling in herself; that this feeling is represented by the dogs (something fierce and not under her control); and that she has to arrange her life so that she avoids not only the dogs, but also any situation in which these feelings might be aroused (which included therapy and especially group therapy).

F. EVIDENCE REQUIRED IN ASSESSMENT OF 'IDEAL' RESULT

(a) Loss of phobia, accompanied by

(b) loss of need to control people and situations so that everyone is nice and kind; and

(c) freedom with her sexual and aggressive feelings.

G. THERAPEUTIC PLAN FORMULATED AT INITIAL ASSESSMENT

After the projection test, which suggested a severe hysterical illness with rigid defences, this patient was regarded as unsuitable for brief psychotherapy. She was therefore offered a preliminary appointment to discuss group treatment, which she failed to keep. She wrote saying she could not face group treatment. She was then offered, and she accepted, brief psychotherapy by the therapist whose group she was due to attend, with the limited aim of enabling her to accept group treatment.

H. SUMMARY OF COURSE OF THERAPY

Session 2 was taken up with her resentment against the original interviewer, who had not been nice and kind to her. In session 3 the therapist forcefully interpreted that her life problem was difficulty in facing her anger, so that she avoided anything which represents anger (such as dogs) and anything which might make her angry (such as unkind therapists or the group). She ended by saying 'I know that the group represents life, and it must be my

(*The dog lady—continued*)

object to go'. After session 5 she agreed to attend the group, which she did twice, sitting tense and rigid and hardly able to say a word. She finally refused to attend any more and returned to individual therapy. In subsequent sessions a peculiar transference situation developed, in which she had to sit with her back to the therapist in order to confess some sexual secret—which in fact she never succeeded in doing. Deadlock. Therapy was then terminated because of the therapist's departure from the clinic.

WORK ON TERMINATION. Although the main focus was the patient's feelings about joining a group, no work was recorded on her feelings about leaving individual therapy.

Total no of sessions   10
Total time   5 months

I. CHANGES IN ALL DISTURBANCES LISTED UNDER C

At termination of individual therapy:

Almost certainly no changes in:

(a) dog phobia, or
(b) need to control external situations, but
(d) terror of group treatment was sufficiently reduced for her to accept group treatment once more, and attend for treatment in two different groups for 3½ years.

There was, however:

(c) much acting out over attendance at the group during this period. She finally left the group in a state of great anxiety, after speaking for the first time of phantasies about the therapist's sexual relation with another woman. Finally, 4 years 3 months after the original termination, she asked for individual therapy in private, but when there was some delay over offering her an appointment she refused to come. Changes at this point are not clear but must be minimal.

J. SUMMARY OF CHANGES. PSYCHODYNAMIC ASSESSMENT OF RESULT

It is clear that the original limited aim, to enable her to attend group treatment, was partly achieved. This is not regarded as a valid therapeutic aim for the purposes of this study.

No score.

K. STATUS OF THE EVIDENCE

Unequivocal.

THE DRAPER'S ASSISTANT

A. DETAILS OF PATIENT AND THERAPIST

1. *Patient*

Sex	F
Age	21
Marital status	Married
Occupation	Assistant in a draper's shop.
Complaint	Fear of sexual intercourse.
What seems to bring patient now	Has been married seven months. Marriage still not consummated.

2. *Therapist*

Code	A
Sex	F

B. PSYCHIATRIC HISTORY AND DIAGNOSIS

Family history. NAD

Home atmosphere. Father tended to get angry and shout.

Menstrual history. FMP at 13. Regular 5/28–29. Very little pain.

Physical examination. Examined at birth control clinic. Introitus admitted three fingers; cervix pointed downwards and forwards; uterus small. No physical reason why she should not have intercourse. (State of hymen not recorded.)

Medical history. No serious illnesses.

Present illness. Husband, seen by us, claimed to be fully potent. Patient is not afraid of childbirth.

Diagnosis. Frigidity and mild phobic anxiety (see below) in an immature personality.

C. ALL KNOWN DISTURBANCES IN PATIENT'S LIFE

Known at initial assessment:

(a) *Sex*
Has never allowed her husband to penetrate properly (though there was a small amount of blood on one occasion, and it is possible her hymen is ruptured). Gets the feeling that she is 'going to burst open' if she allows penetration.

(b) *Phobias*
As long as she can remember she has been afraid
    (i) of being alone in the house, in case a burglar should come in;

77

   (ii) of being alone in the street, in case a man should follow her
       and attack her;
   (iii) of climbing ladders.
None of these fears, however, has ever played a big part in her
life; and none has ever prevented her from doing anything that
she wanted to do.

D. AREAS OF PATIENT'S LIFE UNAFFECTED BY ABOVE DISTURBANCES
(a) Has had a number of boy friends before her husband and has
    erotic feelings when kissed.
(b) Has taken a good deal of responsibility in helping her mother
    at home.

E. MINIMUM PSYCHODYNAMIC HYPOTHESIS SUGGESTED TO EXPLAIN C
Anxiety about her own primitive sexuality.

F. EVIDENCE REQUIRED IN ASSESSMENT OF 'IDEAL' RESULT
(a) She should allow her husband full penetration, without
    anxiety, with enjoyment, with orgasm.
(b) The above should be accompanied by disappearance of her
    phobias.

G. THERAPEUTIC PLAN FORMULATED AT INITIAL ASSESSMENT
No definite plan was made.

H. SUMMARY OF COURSE OF THERAPY
In session 1 this very unsophisticated young woman seemed to
the therapist to be 'trying to have a grown-up conversation about
a part of her that is still a little girl—only no one must say openly
that there is a little girl'.
   It is very difficult to know exactly what happened in this therapy.
Important moments seem to have been:
   (i) Session 2: therapist interpreted patient's fears of having
       her body spoiled. At the end of this session the patient
       warmed up and said, 'It is better to be able to talk to some-
       body'.
   (ii) In session 5 the patient seemed to be keeping the therapist
       at bay by chatting, and the therapist interpreted that she
       was *keeping control of her* in the same way as she had to
       control her husband by refusing intercourse.
   (iii) The patient then missed one session, but in the next session
       said that there had been a 'little blood on the sheet' about a

week before. The therapist advised her to investigate her vagina with her fingers.

(iv) In session 8 the patient reported having lost her wedding ring, and the therapist interpreted that she wished to throw away her marriage, not to become a woman, and to keep her husband angry. She wept and said she knew the therapist and her husband were right, but they didn't understand how impossible it was for her when the time came.

(v) In session 9 the patient reported having *had intercourse several times*, and treatment was terminated at session 10.

WORK ON TERMINATION. None recorded.

Total no. of sessions   10
Total time   5 months

I. CHANGES IN ALL DISTURBANCES LISTED UNDER C

Follow-up (1) 2½ months:

Says she has 'forgotten her difficulties' and that she and her husband are hoping to start a family soon.

Follow-up (2) 2 years:

The patient admitted under pressure that she had *not really had intercourse properly at all*, although there seems to have been a considerable improvement in her mild phobias.[1] She was taken on for another course of treatment (13 further sessions) without apparent improvement. This is not considered in the present study.

J. SUMMARY OF CHANGES. PSYCHODYNAMIC ASSESSMENT OF RESULTS

No change in sexual disturbances. Considerable improvement in symbolic representation of problem, but this was of little importance in her life.

Score 0.

K. STATUS OF THE EVIDENCE

It is not easy to get at the real truth about sexual problems, especially in a patient of this kind, but the evidence is fairly unequivocal.[2]

[1] Later follow-up showed that the phobias either had not really improved or else had returned later.
[2] Later follow-up showed unequivocally that she did not really have intercourse.

79

THE FALLING SOCIAL WORKER

A. DETAILS OF PATIENT AND THERAPIST

1. *Patient*

Sex	F
Age	27
Marital status	Single
Occupation	Social worker for a hospital.
Complaint	Fears of falling and fainting, ten years.
What seems to bring patient now	Referred by psychiatrist who has treated her on and off for four years. Acute exacerbation after pentothal injection by him—he now has to pass her on.

2. *Therapist*

Code	G
Sex	M

B. PSYCHIATRIC HISTORY AND DIAGNOSIS

Family history. NAD

Childhood home atmosphere. Perhaps over-protective, otherwise happy.

Previous history. NAD

Physical examination. General and neurological examination by referring psychiatrist, NAD.

Diagnosis. Phobic anxiety-hysteria in an obsessional personality.

C. ALL KNOWN DISTURBANCES IN PATIENT'S LIFE

(a) *Phobic symptoms*
Fear of falling and fainting, mainly in hospital meetings, but also in the street.

(b) *Relations with men*
Gets herself 'picked up' by disreputable men whom she despises, with whom she has sexual relations short of intercourse. Seeks final satisfaction in masturbation. Cannot make sexual relations with 'decent' men.

(c) *Relations with father. Problems over being herself and leading her own life*
Cannot free herself from her 70-year-old father, who is possessive and jealous of her boy friends. Has always lived at home or in a women's hostel. Has a constant feeling of unreality.

(d) *Compulsive phenomena*

Piles work and responsibility on herself and leaves scarcely any time for other activities.

D. AREAS OF PATIENT'S LIFE UNAFFECTED BY ABOVE DISTURBANCES

(a) Efficient and enthusiastic social worker.
(b) Good capacity for friendship with women.
(c) Uninhibited intellectual curiosity and satisfaction.
(d) Copes well with responsibility.

E. MINIMUM PSYCHODYNAMIC HYPOTHESIS REQUIRED TO EXPLAIN C

Severe conflict over her sexual feelings, which are felt to be forbidden and dirty. The phobias are assumed to represent a symbolic expression of this conflict. Defends herself against the conflict by splitting men into (i) disreputable men for whom she can have sexual feelings, and (ii) 'decent' men for whom she can't. This problem probably has its origins in sexual and other conflicting feelings for her father, with whom she is still deeply involved. Therapy suggested strongly that her feeling of unreality expressed her inability to be herself, because of her feeling that she had to be what other people, especially her father, required her to be.

F. EVIDENCE REQUIRED IN ASSESSMENT OF 'IDEAL' RESULT

(a) Loss of symptoms.
(b) (i) Gives up relations with disreputable men.
    (ii) Able to have sexual feelings for marriageable men.
       Ultimately marriage and enjoyment of sexual intercourse.
(c) Ability to lead her own life—to give up living in girls' hostel and to give up concern for father's jealous attitude to her boy friends. Loss of sense of unreality.
(d) Reduction in compulsive work.

G. THERAPEUTIC PLAN FORMULATED AT INITIAL ASSESSMENT

Not clearly formulated.

H. SUMMARY OF COURSE OF THERAPY

At interview this patient gave the impression of being at different times a middle-aged spinster, a little girl, flirtatious, and sincerely attempting to be forthright and honest. She formed a strong relationship with the therapist at once, and by session 3 this transference had become frankly dependent and with a sexual tinge. The therapist responded by setting her a time limit of three months.

The following foci can be selected from a long and complex therapy:

(i) Inability to accept her own 'bad' feelings (first interpreted in session 1).

(ii) Dependent sexual transference to present therapist (touched on in sessions 1 and 2, partially interpreted in session 3, broke through with a vivid sexual phantasy about therapist in session 10); sexual transference to previous therapist (interpreted in sessions 1 and 4, and thoroughly explored in session 10).

(iii) Difficulty in becoming a woman, related to Oedipal problems (e.g. session 4).

(iv) Conflicting identification with parents; identification with what people (including therapist) require of her, leading to loss of sense of identity (sessions 5–6). This symptom began to improve after this interpretation.

WORK ON TERMINATION AND TEMPORARY ABSENCE. Anticipation of grief at termination was first interpreted in session 1. Feelings about therapist's temporary absence were interpreted in session 8. Anger at the therapist's indifference during the patient's absence through a physical illness was interpreted with a clear response in about session 30; and it then quickly emerged that the patient had always been infuriated by her mother's indifference and coldness. Anger and grief at termination, with defence of manic denial, were made the main focus during about the last ten sessions, and a good deal of open feeling was brought out.

$$\text{Total no. of sessions} \quad 40$$
$$\text{Total time} \quad \quad \quad \quad \text{4 months}$$

I. CHANGES IN ALL DISTURBANCES LISTED UNDER C

Follow-up (1) 1 year 7 months:

(*a*) *Phobic symptoms*. These at first disappeared, but have recently returned. They worry her less than when she came for treatment.

(*b*) *Relations with men*. (i) She says she has no urge towards the 'pick-up' relations with disreputable men any more. Some evidence, however, was obtained from an independent source that she tended to associate with such men at a club which she attended. (ii) She now has two 'marriageable' boy friends, with one of whom she has an intense sexual relation short of inter-course.

(*d*) *Compulsive phenomena.* Gets away from work on time and does not seek extra responsibilities.

Follow-up (2) 3 years (letter from patient):

(*a*) *Phobic symptoms.* 'The only remaining symptom is the fear of meetings . . . although it persists it doesn't worry me any more.'

(*b*) *Relations with men.* Her relation with one boy friend came to an end when he gave her an ultimatum that either she slept with him or they parted, and she chose the latter. She now has another boy friend, and says that she is starting a 'new "friendship" based for the first time not on physical attraction so much as our affection and common interests. I am not in love, but I am happy.'

(*c*) *Ability to lead her own life.* 'I know who I am and I know what I want, and I don't live in a dream-world any more.'

(*d*) *Compulsive phenomena.* 'Work is far less interesting than formerly, and I could easily give it up if I had a home to run. I do not volunteer to do any extras.'

J. SUMMARY OF CHANGES. PSYCHODYNAMIC ASSESSMENT OF RESULT

(a) Reduction in symptoms.
(b) Inappropriate reaction to men substantially replaced by appropriate reaction, though probably leaving residual sexual inhibitions.
(c) Inability to be herself and live her own life replaced by appropriate reaction.
(d) Disappearance of compulsive work.

Though not a complete success—one would like to see her happily married—a very substantial improvement.

Score 3.

K. STATUS OF THE EVIDENCE

Although the final follow-up was based only on a letter, this letter was full and frank, and the evidence is almost unequivocal.

THE GIRL WITH THE DREAMS

A. DETAILS OF PATIENT AND THERAPIST

1. *Patient*

Sex	F
Age	24
Marital status	Single
Occupation	Assistant to an estate manager.
Complaint	Difficulty in concentration, lack of confidence, frightening dreams (a few years).
What seems to bring patient now	Two months ago she had a severe panic attack in which she thought she was going to have a fit.

2 *Therapist*

Code	A
Sex	F

B. PSYCHIATRIC HISTORY AND DIAGNOSIS

Family history. Father had some sort of nervous breakdown many years ago, details not known. Two female cousins: one believed to be epileptic, one schizophrenic.

Home atmosphere. Patient remembers her childhood as happy, but she had little contact with her mother.

Previous history. In her teens she had a panic attack in which she 'thought there was a knife in her hand and that she wanted to kill her mother', although there was no knife in her hand in fact.

Menstrual history. FMP at 14, regular 3/26

Medical history. No serious illnesses. No convulsions.

Physical examination. GP (an ex-psychiatrist) reported a general and physical examination NAD.

Present illness. The details of the recent attack were as follows: She was in her room one evening with her fiancé, when she suddenly became severely anxious, 'went stiff with fright', lay down, and lay twitching all over for several minutes. The twitching started in her shoulders, where she had been experiencing tension (see below). No disturbance of consciousness or incontinence.

Diagnosis. Anxiety-hysteria with obsessional features. In view of the clear history of neurotic disturbance and the typical hysterical

84

features, the diagnosis of epilepsy was considered unlikely and she was not given an EEG.

C. ALL KNOWN DISTURBANCES IN PATIENT'S LIFE

1. Known at initial interview:

Has suffered from the following for a number of years:

(a) *Symptoms*

(i) *Anxiety*: seems to be frightened about something most of the time. Perspires a lot, and feels tension in the scapular region. *Vivid and rather frightening dreams*, the main theme of which is *having to cross a bridge with the sea on either side.*

(ii) More severe *panic attacks* from time to time, in some of which she is afraid something awful may happen to someone (e.g. her mother or her fiancé). The worst was the recent one (see B above).

(iii) *Obsessional phenomena* (not severe): e.g. if she has pulled the lavatory plug she has to be a certain way away before the water stops rushing, or has to cross a street in a certain way; otherwise she has the feeling that something awful may happen to someone.

(iv) *General*: difficulty in concentration. Lack of confidence. Dreams things and can't remember whether they were dreams or reality.

(b) *Difficulty over anger—Relation to women*

She can't answer people back, particularly women (and probably including her mother) and may spend a long time going over in her mind all the things she would have liked to say.

2. Which came to light during therapy:

(c) *Sexual problems*

Feels sexual intercourse is wrong unless it is in order to have a baby. Is always left with a strong feeling of dissatisfaction afterwards. Feels safer with less masculine men.

D. AREAS OF PATIENT'S LIFE UNAFFECTED BY ABOVE DISTURBANCES

Has managed to do well in the externals of life.

E. MINIMUM PSYCHODYNAMIC HYPOTHESIS SUGGESTED TO EXPLAIN C

The problem is somewhat complex and seems to contain the following elements:

(i) Guilt and anxiety over becoming a woman. Probably guilt about rivalry with women, including her mother. The sea

85

(The girl with the dreams—continued)

in the dreams may at least in part represent sexuality and femininity.

(ii) Guilt and anxiety over aggressive feelings towards both sexes. The panic attack may well represent her fear of losing control.

F. EVIDENCE REQUIRED IN ASSESSMENT OF 'IDEAL' RESULT

(a) Loss of all symptoms—frightening dreams, panic attacks, obsessional symptoms, lack of concentration, etc.

(b) and (c):

    (i) Ability to accept her femininity and enjoy a satisfactory relation with a man, including a sexual relation.

    (ii) Ability to form a satisfactory relation with women, especially older women, and including her mother.

    (iii) Satisfactory relation with her baby (see below).

    (iv) No longer anxious about her anger. Able to control it but to express it freely where appropriate.

G. THERAPEUTIC PLAN FORMULATED AT INITIAL ASSESSMENT

This was not specifically stated, but by implication was to show her how her disturbed relationship with her mother was interfering with her acceptance of femininity.

H. SUMMARY OF COURSE OF THERAPY

The patient arrived at the first session with her therapist (session 2) dressed in jeans, looking like 'an adolescent pretty boy'. After some slight initial difficulty she formed an easy relation, and was able to speak quite intimately about her feelings.

Therapy was sharply divided into two phases: sessions 1–8 almost entirely non-transference; and sessions 9–18 in which transference interpretations became important. In the first phase work was done on the patient's feelings of disgust for bodies and sexuality, resentment against her mother and men, and difficulties over accepting femininity. Early in this phase the patient, who was unmarried, told the therapist that she was pregnant. The wedding took place during a six-week break between sessions 8 and 9. When she told her parents that she was already pregnant they took it very well.

Perhaps the most striking and most hopeful material came in the first session after her marriage (session 9), a dream on the usual theme of the sea but with a much more reassuring ending: *a woman was let down into a stormy sea; it was the patient's turn next, and she was relieved to find that the woman was unharmed.*

The therapist interpreted herself—a woman who had already accepted femininity—as the woman in the dream, with the implication that this marked the beginning of the patient's acceptance of femininity, and the reconciliation with the therapist as mother. In later sessions much further work was done on dreams. Interpretations were made about sexual feelings for the patient's father and brother; about the feeling that she had no right to her baby, and that the therapist or her mother would take it away from her out of jealousy; and the feeling that in order to have her baby, therefore, she must kill the therapist or her mother. Most of these interpretations were based on very clear material, and the patient understood and accepted them.

WORK ON TERMINATION. In sessions 15, 17, and 18 there were interpretations about termination. The patient responded with open grief. A single recorded interpretation about anger over termination met with a doubtful response.

Total no. of sessions   18
Total time   8 months

I. CHANGES IN ALL DISTURBANCES LISTED UNDER C

1. At termination (independent assessment):

(*a*) *Symptoms.* The dreams are less frightening. They are mainly concerned with her baby, but are not entirely reassuring—e.g. she dreams that she has not experienced the birth, the baby is already six months old, and it seems that her mother has more or less had it for her. No information about the other symptoms.

(*b*) and (*c*):

(i) She has married the father of her child. Information about their relation is scanty.

(ii) She seems to have become reconciled to her mother. 'Now we have something in common. She's a mother and I'm a mother.' She says that both parents have recently been able to talk more freely about their feelings for her, which has helped her a lot, because they used to be so undemonstrative.

(iii) Anger: no information.

(*d*) *Emergence of new problem—depression.* Both independent interviewer and psychologist who re-tested her felt that she was now depressed—though this also meant that she seemed a much deeper person than before.

2. Follow-up, 7 months (and including information obtained during second phase of therapy):

87

(The girl with the dreams—continued)

(*a*) *Symptoms. Dreams*: no longer so frightening. *Panic attacks*: had at least one before final termination, but has never twitched or lost consciousness. *Obsessional symptoms*: no evidence. *Confusion between phantasy and reality*: unchanged.

(*b*) and (*c*):

(i) *Relation with husband*: she feels her husband is weak, her physical response to him is limited, and she is still left with a sense of dissatisfaction after intercourse.

(ii) *Relation with mother*: reconciliation seems maintained, though information is meagre. Mother was very enthusiastic about the baby, even though it was conceived out of wedlock.

(iii) *Relation with baby*: this seems to be entirely satisfactory. She breast-fed him, and he gives very little trouble.

(iv) *Anger*: no information.

(*d*) *Depression*. No longer seems depressed, though she seems muddled.

3. Second course of therapy:

Patient was now taken on for a second course of therapy, successfully terminated after a total of 8 sessions. During this period her husband was also taken on for brief psychotherapy by another therapist. This further course of treatment did not result in any unequivocal further changes, and is not considered in the present study.

J. SUMMARY OF CHANGES. PSYCHODYNAMIC ASSESSMENT OF RESULT

This is an extremely difficult assessment. The agreed but highly inferential opinion of the Workshop was that she had largely solved her problem in relation to women and to being a mother, but that the problem in relation to men was essentially unchanged. Absence of solution to the heterosexual problem prevents a score of 3. Evidence of improvement in one problem of human relations makes the score higher than 1.

Tentative score, therefore, 2.

K. STATUS OF THE EVIDENCE

Unsatisfactory:

(i) because the second course of therapy obscures further follow-up and

(ii) because this was a therapy in which many of the changes have to be inferred from rather intangible evidence.

THE HYPERTENSIVE HOUSEWIFE

A. DETAILS OF PATIENT AND THERAPIST

1. Patient

Sex	F
Age	34
Marital status	Married
Occupation	Housewife
Complaint	Headaches, bad dreams, uncontrollable outbursts.
What seems to bring patient now	Fear that her outbursts are affecting her children, since her return to her husband two months ago. Her GP has been treating her with psychotherapy and needs help.

2. Therapist

Code	D
Sex	M

B. PSYCHIATRIC HISTORY AND DIAGNOSIS

Family history. Mother died eleven years ago of high blood pressure. Two members of mother's family also died of high blood pressure.

Home atmosphere. Father tyrannical; mother had violent outbursts of temper.

Medical history. Suffered from high blood pressure during several pregnancies.

Diagnosis. Severe reactive depression with anxiety.

C. ALL KNOWN DISTURBANCES IN PATIENT'S LIFE

(a) *Symptoms*
Headaches and a feeling of pressure on top of her head. Bad dreams, some of them about violence.

(b) *Tendency to have relations with disturbed men*
She originally married a man who, though kind to her, seems to be physically and emotionally ill, which she did not know at the time. He suffers from a severe eczema on his body, for which he refuses treatment, and she is repelled by him. She now refuses any sexual relation with him but probably also resents his lack of aggression.

89

(The hypertensive housewife—continued)

At the beginning of their marriage he often masturbated in half-sleep. She has one child by him.

Nine years ago she left her husband and went to live with a man with whom she was very happy, and by whom she had two children. He was violent and sometimes threw knives at her. He fell ill, they got into financial difficulties and he used to steal. He finally died four years ago. She returned to her husband two months ago.

(c) *Depressive manifestations*

She never got over the death of her lover four years ago, became depressed and irritable, and two years ago made a suicidal attempt with tablets. She began to eat very little. At interview she spent her whole time turned away from the interviewer, wringing her hands. The psychologist described her as 'very acutely depressed' and 'giving the impression of extreme tension'. The therapist described her as 'retarded'.

(d) *Manifest aggressiveness*

Uncontrollable outbursts of temper.

D. AREAS OF PATIENT'S LIFE UNAFFECTED BY ABOVE DISTURBANCES

None known.

E. MINIMUM PSYCHODYNAMIC HYPOTHESIS REQUIRED TO EXPLAIN C

These disturbances can all be explained on the basis of a severe conflict over her own aggressiveness. She has alternated between a man who is not aggressive with whom her relation is unsatisfactory, and a man who is violent with whom she says she was happy. While her outbursts express her violence, her depression is assumed to express her guilt about it.

F. EVIDENCE REQUIRED IN ASSESSMENT OF 'IDEAL' RESULT

There should be evidence that she no longer suffers from uncontrollable outbursts, but is able to express anger effectively when it is appropriate to do so. Her depression should disappear permanently. A satisfactory solution of her problem over men seems hardly possible in the circumstances, but some sort of tolerable compromise should be reached.

G. THERAPEUTIC PLAN FORMULATED AT INITIAL ASSESSMENT

Balint: '3–6 months, to allow her to accept her hatred and not push it onto other people.'

H. SUMMARY OF COURSE OF THERAPY

The original interview was very difficult, since the patient apparently had difficulty in hearing what the interviewer said. This difficulty disappeared temporarily but dramatically when the interviewer interpreted that nothing could be done for her unless it was possible to get in touch with the wicked part of her. In session 3 and several subsequent sessions, the therapist tried to get her to look at her 'wicked self'—e.g. her resentment at the way the doctors had neglected her lover who died—without apparent success. In session 7 the patient began to talk much more freely about herself and her childhood: e.g. telling of her mother's bad tempers and lack of sympathy; of her mother's death (eleven years ago), and the fact that her father forced her (the patient) to lay out her mother's body, which she deeply resented; of the fact that she (the patient) had been told that she could not have further children because of high blood pressure, which also ran in the family and of which her mother had died; that nevertheless her lover had refused to use contraceptives, and as a result she had had to have three abortions. The therapist pointed out her tremendous preoccupation with the death of people near to her, and suggested that *she feared that her own destructive impulses had killed them. After this session she said she felt considerable relief.* Work continued on her resentment and destructiveness, and signs of a *desire for reparative activities* began to appear in her. She volunteered as a blood donor, was visiting a blind woman, and went to a First Aid course. She also went to the hospital to get a hearing aid. In session 13 she said that she was far less depressed; and that she had decided to try and live her life with her husband, but as independently as possible. By session 17 she had persuaded her husband to come to see the therapist, which he did. He was very pleased with his wife's improvement, but he refused to seek treatment for his eczema (he did in fact do so some time later). Therapy was terminated by mutual agreement after session 19.

WORK ON TERMINATION. None recorded.

Total no. of sessions 19
Total time 6 months

Subsequent events:

She was then seen for independent assessment by the original interviewer. In this interview she was extremely cheerful and approachable until the sexual relation with her husband was discussed, and it then emerged that she had consistently refused

(The hypertensive housewife—continued)

any sexual contact with him. She then became very tense and fidgety. She felt that the interviewer conveyed to her that until she could accept sexual intercourse she could not be regarded as improved. She was seen again by the therapist one week later, full of despair and resentment, and *feeling that things were as bad as ever.* She was taken on again and therapy became long-term. After a total of 39 sessions she had to be admitted to a neurosis unit because of depression. When the time came for her discharge from there she took a small overdose of tablets and was transferred to a mental hospital. According to our latest information (one year after final termination) she was now better, was due for discharge, and was intending to leave her husband and get a job.

I. SUMMARY OF CHANGES. PSYCHODYNAMIC ASSESSMENT OF RESULT

Marked improvement in headaches and depressive symptoms, followed by immediate relapse.

Score 0.

J. STATUS OF THE EVIDENCE

Unequivocal.

THE LIGHTERMAN

A. DETAILS OF PATIENT AND THERAPIST

1. *Patient*

Sex	M
Age	30
Marital status	Married
Occupation	Lighterman on the Thames.
Complaint	Severe anxiety attacks, two months.
What seems to bring patient now	Developed these attacks soon after a minor accident to his barge, in which he was hit on the head but not seriously injured.

2. *Therapist*

Code	F
Sex	M

B. PSYCHIATRIC HISTORY AND DIAGNOSIS

Family history. Mother is severely compulsive in a similar way to patient. She had a breakdown lasting three years when the patient was 4 or 5, in which she thought people were talking about her. One brother compulsive also.

Previous personality. Not unduly anxious, but somewhat hypochondriacal.

Medical history. Previous head injury at 13, with fracture of base of skull. Uneventful recovery. No sequelae. No other serious illnesses.

Present illness. (i) During at least the last seven years the compulsive phenomena described below have been present. (ii) 4/12 ago he took a decision to emigrate, but when there was delay over formalities he began to get increasingly tense and irritable. (iii) 2/12 ago his barge was involved in a collision and he was struck on the head by the tiller. He was not knocked out and there was no amnesia, but he was dazed for a short time. Two days later he had the first of his severe anxiety attacks accompanied by confusion; and later there developed increased irritability, headaches, depression, intolerance of noise, and phobias.

Physical examination. Owing to an oversight, this patient was never physically examined.

Diagnosis. Since his injury this man has suffered from many of the symptoms of the well-recognized 'post-traumatic syndrome',

93

together with more obviously psychoneurotic symptoms such as depression and phobias. Until recently there has been considerable doubt about the extent of organic factors in this syndrome, but the work of Dencker (1958) on twins strongly suggests that the syndrome is entirely psychogenic with a strong constitutional element.

The diagnosis is therefore as follows: a patient suffering from a moderately severe compulsive neurosis who, after a relatively trivial head injury, showed a post-traumatic syndrome which was probably entirely psychogenic. The manifestations of neurosis after head injury were severe anxiety attacks, phobic anxiety, and mild reactive depression.

C. ALL KNOWN DISTURBANCES IN PATIENT'S LIFE

1. Background problems:

(a) *Compulsive phenomena* (gradually increasing over last few years)
It is not easy to give an impression of the extent to which this man's life was affected by compulsiveness, because all the things that he felt compelled to do were in themselves perfectly 'normal'. The difference from 'normality' lay in the degree of tension which he suffered if he failed to give in to his compulsions.

At work he often feels compelled to write down even the simplest instructions to make sure he's got it all right. Unable to refuse overtime. As a result, grossly overworks, earning £20–25 a week. If his departure is delayed he has to find some other job to do. At home has to be constantly occupied. Feels compelled to finish any job at once—e.g. if the toaster goes wrong he has to mend it before breakfast. Feels compelled to go to bed early and get up early. If his wife is preparing a meal feels compelled to help her.

(b) *Relation with mother*
Considerably affected by compulsiveness. Feels compelled to visit her as often as his wife can be persuaded to go—two or three times a week.

2. Breakdown into acute anxiety following mild head injury:

(c) *Severe anxiety and confusional attacks*
Has had about three. Feels that his head is in a jumble, that he will pass out; once wrote his name and address on a bit of paper in case he was picked up unconscious.

94

(d) *Less severe anxiety and confusional states*
These, which may last for days, are set off by situations of anger, delay, conflict, noise: e.g. in traffic jams, when a wireless blares, at football matches. He has had a row with a neighbour and feels tense whenever he gets home.

(e) *Relations with his children*
If they make a noise, are naughty, or make demands on him, he loses his temper. He has thrashed his son on several occasions.

3. The following developed during the therapy period:

(f) *Phobias*
Complicated mixture of agoraphobia and claustrophobia. Cannot take his barge into the open river but feels all right in the docks. His employer has adjusted his work accordingly. Yet he also has a fear of enclosed spaces, and likes to be driven by his wife into the country in his car. Does not like travelling alone on trains.

(g) *Depressive phenomena*
Crying attacks, suicidal thoughts, fear that he may commit suicide.

D. AREAS OF PATIENT'S LIFE UNAFFECTED BY ABOVE DISTURBANCES

Apparently has an extremely good relation with his wife, who is tolerant and understanding and looks after him.

E. MINIMUM PSYCHODYNAMIC HYPOTHESIS SUGGESTED TO EXPLAIN C

Uppermost seems to be a severe problem over aggression. Therapy suggested that this was mainly anger with his mother. The anxiety probably represents his fear of being overwhelmed by aggressive impulses, the obsessional phenomena his defence against them and his guilt about them.

F. EVIDENCE REQUIRED IN ASSESSMENT OF 'IDEAL' RESULT

Loss of all the above symptoms. Ability to control his aggression, but to be aggressive in an effective way when the situation demands it. There should be no restrictions such as those imposed by his phobias.

G. THERAPEUTIC PLAN FORMULATED AT INITIAL ASSESSMENT

To give him insight into what happened inside him when he had the accident.

H. SUMMARY OF COURSE OF THERAPY

This fine, strong working-class man, whose bewildered distress and genuine desire for insight made everybody very keen to help him, was first seen for an ORT. During this he de-repressed the memory of a previous incident which had been traumatic for him (a *road accident* to a little girl that he had witnessed some years before). As a result of this he arrived at the initial interview (immediately after the ORT) in a *confusional state*. The observable manifestation of this was that, talking under great pressure, he changed rapidly from one subject to another, mixing up several different—though always related—themes in an apparently random manner, so that it was not easy to follow him. He was unable to talk about this traumatic memory and the interview was marked by a lack of communication. Non-transference interpretations of the patient's guilt about being selfish, though clearly indicated, had no effect. In session 3 the therapist converted these into a transference interpretation, suggesting that the patient was afraid of being criticized by the therapist, as by his father, for being a nuisance to his mother. The patient (who had recovered from his confusional state) at once *became confused once more*, and from this confusion the story of the *accident to the little girl* finally emerged. This led, during sessions 4-14, to non-transference work about the patient's childhood conflict with his mother, resulting in the expression of a great deal of anger against her. She had told him that he was an unwanted child and had shown excessive anxiety about his *playing in the road*—presumably in order to defend herself against her wish to get rid of him. During this period three links were made: those between his mother's anxiety over his playing in the road and

(i) the accident to the little girl, which the patient partially accepted;

(ii) the patient's own accident (the precipitating cause of his anxiety attacks), which the patient surprisingly never accepted; and

(iii) the phobia of going into the open *river*, which the patient accepted with enthusiasm but which had no effect upon this phobia at all.

WORK ON TERMINATION AND TEMPORARY ABSENCE. After session 10 the therapist had to move away and an attempt at termination was made. Four months later the therapist asked to see the patient who arrived in a state of anxiety and mild confusion. This was resolved when the patient was finally enabled to *criticize the therapist* for not having already known (in session 3) about the accident to the little girl—about which the patient had told the psychologist just before session 1. The link was made to the patient's anger with his mother for not looking after him properly. The patient was then allowed to space the sessions himself. In session 15 there was further anxiety, relieved by bringing out further criticism. In sessions 16 and 17 the patient reported marked anxiety and acting out away from the session, relieved by interpretations about his need to have the therapist 'on tap', his guilt about this, and his anger when the therapist was not available.

Total no. of sessions   17
Total time   15 months

I. CHANGES IN ALL DISTURBANCES LISTED UNDER C

Follow-up (1) 1 year 7 months:

(*a*) *Compulsive phenomena.* Now does not do much overtime and is perfectly content to earn £14 a week. Does not feel compelled to do jobs around the house at once—'my wife says I'm getting quite lazy'. Less compelled to check things at work. Still not happy unless he can occupy himself, but has replaced tensely compulsive activities by activities which may still be somewhat compulsive but are more in the nature of 'reparation', e.g. has taken to mending shoes as a hobby and has taken an orphan into his home.

(*b*) *Relation with mother.* Has 'had it out' with her and their relation has considerably improved. She has discussed his childhood with him. He now no longer feels compelled to visit her, and goes once a week or once a fortnight.

(*c*) and (*d*) *Acute and chronic anxiety and confusion.* Has had no severe anxiety attacks. He still gets somewhat tense in some of the same situations as before, but instead of lasting for days this rarely lasts more than a quarter of an hour. He is able to control it by doing something else, and on at least two occasions to disperse it by analysing his own feelings.

(*e*) *Relations with his children.* Because he works less overtime now he sees them almost every night, and the relation with them has enormously improved. He reads to them and lets them climb all over him. He copes realistically with their demands for more— 'just one more story and then up to bed'. When they are naughty

97

The present work

(The lighterman—continued)

he deals with them firmly and sends his son off to bed instead of
thrashing him.

(*f*) *Phobias.* These remain *largely unchanged.* He still gets anxious
when closed in, and would not like to travel by train. He refuses
to go back to the open river, saying he never liked the job, and it
looks as if he could not go back if he tried.

(*g*) *Depressive phenomena.* These have not recurred.

Follow-up (2) 4 years (letter from patient):

Patient writes: '. . . as I am now so much better I do not feel I
want to visit you [*sic*] clinic, hoping I do not sound ungrateful,
thank you for what you did for me.'

J. SUMMARY OF CHANGES. PSYCHODYNAMIC ASSESSMENT OF RESULT

(a) Anxiety attacks largely replaced by phobias.
(b) Marked replacement of compulsive by reparative activities
which—though still perhaps somewhat compulsive—are much
less anxiety-laden and can bring some satisfaction.
(c) Some ability to express anger appropriately instead of having
an 'all or nothing' reaction. Consequent great improvement in
the relation with his mother and with his children.

A very complex result, in which the favourable changes are
spoiled by the development of the phobias. The final refusal of
follow-up probably indicates the patient's realization that his
position is unstable. Very difficult to assess.

On balance, score 3.

K. STATUS OF THE EVIDENCE

In view of the above, doubtful.

THE NEURASTHENIC'S HUSBAND

A. DETAILS OF PATIENT AND THERAPIST

1. *Patient*

Sex — M
Age — Over 50
Marital status — Married
Occupation — Mathematician working for an industrial firm.
Complaint — Inability to deal with his wife.
What seems to bring patient now — See B below.

2. *Therapist*

Code — E
Sex — M

B. PSYCHIATRIC HISTORY AND DIAGNOSIS

Family history. One sister very neurotic, withdrawn, used to threaten suicide.

Present illness. About fifteen years ago he applied for psychoanalysis, complaining mainly of fear of impotence. He was put on the waiting list but never offered a vacancy, although he did later have about a year's psychotherapy. One year ago he wrote to the Institute complaining of a severe resistance against doing anything but the barest minimum, and a feeling of oppression about all the things left undone. Finally he wrote to the Tavistock Clinic saying that, since his wife had been admitted to hospital, he had experienced a sudden upsurge of energy; and he felt that this was an important opportunity for psychotherapy.

Diagnosis. Life-long neurotic character disorder; chronic depression, now spontaneously lifting. The depression is probably reactive to the failure of his relation with his wife.

C. ALL KNOWN DISTURBANCES IN PATIENT'S LIFE

All come under the heading of a lifelong inability to *assert himself*:

(a) *Relations with wife and women in general*
He regards women as powerful creatures who cannot be criticized and must be placated. His wife is a very disturbed person who has suffered from psychosomatic complaints for many years, and has

99

been under the constant care of a woman doctor. He idealizes his wife's treatment and feels envious of it. He is quite unable to deal with his wife, behaves as a slave to her needs, does not think of his own needs at all, and feels constant resentment at this. He has intercourse only when he feels she wants it, and when he does he cannot satisfy her. He seeks his own satisfaction in masturbation. He submits to her in the house, does the woman's chores, does what she tells him. He does not know whether he can stand her any longer or whether he can do without her. He feels like a small boy, unhappy and despairing.

(b) *Relations at work*
Although he is good at his work he is extremely self-depreciatory in his relations with colleagues and superiors. He allows himself to be paid at far less than his true value. He feels insecure, regards himself as lucky to have the job, and is always afraid he may lose it.

(c) *Relations with children*
He feels his children have no respect for him. In fact they consult his wife rather than him.

D. AREAS OF PATIENT'S LIFE UNAFFECTED BY ABOVE DISTURBANCES

None known. His life as a husband, father, mathematician, employee, as well as his social life—all are affected.

E. MINIMUM PSYCHODYNAMIC HYPOTHESIS REQUIRED TO EXPLAIN C

Since in this case all known disturbances come under the heading of inability to assert himself, there is no need for a psychodynamic hypothesis in the assessment of the result. The hypothesis was made, however, that he had denigrated his father and then felt unable to be more of a man than he. Confirmatory evidence for this was obtained during therapy.

F. EVIDENCE REQUIRED IN ASSESSMENT OF 'IDEAL' RESULT

Evidence that he is able to assert himself, spreading throughout his whole life, e.g.:

(a) *Relation with wife.* Increased potency: ability to serve in intercourse not only his wife's needs but also his own; ability to assert himself in the home, e.g. no longer does the woman's chores, sometimes makes his wife do what he wants, etc. Ability to be angry appropriately and effectively.

(The neurasthenic's husband—continued)

(b) *Relations at work.* Ability to value himself more highly, to be self-seeking and self-assertive, to enjoy taking charge of things.

G. THERAPEUTIC PLAN FORMULATED AT INITIAL ASSESSMENT

Formulated after session 3: 'The immediate aim is to see him two or three times more to see how far interpretation of his identification with his useless father and his anger against women who make him suffer . . . and rule his life will lead him to clearer expression and decision about whether or not he wants his wife back in his home.'

H. SUMMARY OF COURSE OF THERAPY

This patient, a smallish, worried-looking man, started by pouring out a mass of complaints, mournfully, reasonably, with self-contempt and without shame. He showed a great deal of psychological sophistication, and interpretation failed to halt the flood of words or to lead to any fresh insight. The therapist, though initially very pessimistic, persisted with therapy.

The main focus was denigration of his father as useless, identification with his father and the consequent feeling that he himself was useless, the longing for a strong father, and the feeling that women (in contrast to men) were immensely powerful and had to be placated. Manifestations of these feelings in his life outside were interpreted from the beginning, and in the transference from session 2 onwards (e.g. polite denigration of the therapist's remarks, the feeling that patient and therapist together were no match for the patient's wife and her woman doctor, homosexually tinged longing for the therapist and the need to borrow his power). The result was steady but unspectacular progress, with new signs of self-assertiveness both at home and at work.

WORK ON TERMINATION. The climax of therapy came over the question of termination. In session 9 the therapist set a time limit of about 5 more sessions. The patient responded at first by denying that the therapist meant this, and later by saying that there was no sense in coming any more. Interpretations about his fear of being deserted and his defence against this were repeatedly made and met with partial response. In session 13 the interpretation that he was now pretending to be independent to *avoid feelings of longing for a man* (i.e. *a strong father*), as he had done all his life, met with a marked response. The therapist went on to interpret

101

(The neurasthenic's husband—continued)

forcefully that this independence from therapist and father expressed his wish to *deny that therapist and father had any power*, i.e. sexual potency. In session 14 the patient had completely forgotten these interpretations, and similar interpretations had to be repeated. There was again a marked response.

Total no. of sessions 14
Total time 5 months

I. CHANGES IN ALL DISTURBANCES LISTED UNDER C
Follow-up (1) 5 months:

(a) *Relation with wife.* Although the difficulty in dealing with his wife remains, he has been able to assert himself in many ways. He feels no need to submit to her and is often able to handle her in such a way that she does not try to dominate him. He is able to make her do things his way. He no longer does the woman's chores. Sexually he is unable to satisfy her, but he is now able to assert himself better and to attend to his own needs and not only to hers. Masturbation has ceased. He has decided to stay with his wife. He no longer feels in despair, but can accept the limitations of his situation.

(b) *Relations at work.* He remains critical of his work situation but is now not unhappy and can look forward to the future with more reasoned ideas. He has had two large increases in salary, both of which he got by demanding to be paid for what he was worth. He is no longer in fear of losing his job.

(c) *Relations with children.* He now feels that they respect him. In fact his son has recently remarked that the patient has had to bear a great deal of responsibility and has borne it well.

Follow-up (2) 1 year 5 months:

Has obtained another large increase in salary by going in to the managing director and saying he is worth more. He has now himself been made a director. Otherwise hardly any change from previous follow-up.

Follow-up (3) 3 years 3 months:

(a) *Relations with wife and women in general.* His wife has now been told by her doctor that nothing more can be done for her, and she is in a depressed and upset state. He puts up with this as best he can, but is fed up with it, feels he has lost sympathy with her, and sometimes loses his temper. Their sexual relation has

(*The neurasthenic's husband—continued*)

ceased. He is now able to criticize his wife's doctor and her treatment.

(*b*) *Relations at work*. Has recently had a further rise in salary. Patient remarked jokingly that last year he didn't get the rise that he expects just before seeing the therapist, since no appointment was made. Therapist had the impression that he had asked for these increases in salary in a grumbling rather than a self-assertive way. Has a great deal more responsibility than when he started treatment, but there is still room for improvement.

(*c*) *Relations with children*. Improvement maintained.

J. SUMMARY OF CHANGES. PSYCHODYNAMIC ASSESSMENT OF RESULT

Extensive, though by no means complete, replacement of inappropriate by appropriate reaction. Evidence that he still depends on the relation with the therapist for some of his self-confidence, but a 'transference cure' would not be expected to last as long as this.

Score 3.

K. STATUS OF THE EVIDENCE

Satisfactory.

The present work

A. DETAILS OF PATIENT AND THERAPIST

1. *Patient*

Sex	M
Age	28
Marital status	Single
Occupation	Electrical engineer working for a post-graduate degree.
Complaint	Fear that he is homosexual.
What seems to bring patient now	The fear has become so strong that he is afraid he will shout it out at work.

2. *Therapist*

Code	F
Sex	M

B. PSYCHIATRIC HISTORY AND DIAGNOSIS

Family history.
Home atmosphere. } Not fully known.

Previous illnesses. Attack of preoccupation with competition and homosexual feelings five years ago. Seen for psychotherapy for about a year, once a week. Improved. A year or two later suffered a temporary increase of the above symptoms, possibly in a delirious state due to a severe infective illness.

Present illness. Further increase of symptoms, five weeks.

Mental state. He showed traces of most of the signs of paranoid schizophrenia, and yet each was so modified and toned down as to make the diagnosis not quite certain. These included traces of thought disorder; hints of hallucinations that he knew to be hallucinations; delusions that he knew to be delusions; and paranoid ideas that he claimed were reality and really might have been.

Diagnosis. By far the best diagnosis is a man struggling to control paranoid schizophrenia, and aware that he was doing so.

C. ALL KNOWN DISTURBANCES IN PATIENT'S LIFE

(a) *Psychotic thoughts*   (b) *Relations with men*
This man's main symptoms were concerned with internal anxieties about his relations with men. He was perpetually obsessed with a

104

(The paranoid engineer—continued)

comparison between himself and other men, and with a conflict between being active and passive in relation to them. The presence of other men caused him intense anxiety due to the fear that he was homosexual. He had practically all the time to fight down the impulse to shout aloud that he was homosexual. He expressed the fear that after voicing these thoughts to the therapist he wouldn't be able to tell the difference between the clinic and the laboratory, and would voice the same thoughts there.

(c) *Heterosexual problems*
He has fairly strong heterosexual feelings, and has had heterosexual relations in the past, in at least one of which he suffered from premature ejaculation.

D. AREAS OF PATIENT'S LIFE UNAFFECTED BY ABOVE DISTURBANCES

He has managed to graduate and is now studying for a postgraduate degree in engineering. He is working as an engineer at the same time. He manages to hold down his present job without people apparently noticing that there is much wrong with him.

E. MINIMUM PSYCHODYNAMIC HYPOTHESIS SUGGESTED TO EXPLAIN C

No attempt will be made to form a hypothesis about the psychotic nature of this patient's disturbance. The problems in relation to men and women can be explained on the basis of intense anxiety about sexual rivalry with men, with submissive homosexuality as a defence against this.

F. EVIDENCE REQUIRED IN ASSESSMENT OF 'IDEAL' RESULT

(a) Marked reduction in psychotic quality of patient's thoughts.
(b) Ability to form satisfactory relations with men; involving neither excessive competitiveness, nor hostility, nor submissiveness. Ability to fulfil his potential in achievement.
(c) Satisfactory relations with women, including an increase in potency.

G. THERAPEUTIC PLAN FORMULATED AT INITIAL ASSESSMENT

To help to reconcile him to his homosexuality. Therapist had only 7 more sessions available before leaving the clinic.

H. SUMMARY OF COURSE OF THERAPY

At interview this patient showed a psychotic manner, an intense desire to communicate, and an intense fear of doing so, arousing

(The paranoid engineer—continued)

in the therapist a great desire to make contact with him. It was over an hour before the patient dared to speak of his homosexual feelings and problems with men. The next two sessions also largely consisted in helping him to speak about his psychotic thoughts. In session 4, after an interpretation about his feeling of sexual inferiority to the therapist, he had an extremely dramatic psychotic episode in which he seemed to re-live, in the transference, an incident in which he had been homosexually assaulted as a child. After this session therapy was much less intense up to the attempted termination after session 8. He was then seen 2½ months later and, since he continued to ask for help, sessions were continued at irregular intervals. There was another dramatic session (10) in which material about his relations with men led to material and interpretations about childhood competition with his father, fear of killing his father, and the wish to castrate himself. This brought out the memory that as a child he had felt so guilty about masturbation that he had once tried to burn his penis with a red-hot iron. He ended by saying that he felt that his conversation with the therapist had been a sort of fight in which he had proved himself a man.

There was some improvement in his fears about his relations with men, followed by a further attempted termination. He then quickly relapsed and the therapist finally agreed to take him on for long-term treatment. Although this further work was successfully terminated after about 70 sessions in three years with considerable improvements (he passed his post-graduate exams and got married) it is not considered relevant to the present study.

WORK ON TERMINATION. None recorded for the period of therapy considered here.

Total no. of sessions   13 (failure to terminate)
Total time   8 months

I. CHANGES IN ALL DISTURBANCES LISTED UNDER C

None. Failure to terminate.

Score 0.

J. STATUS OF THE EVIDENCE

For the period of therapy considered, failure is clear cut.

THE PILOT'S WIFE

A. DETAILS OF PATIENT AND THERAPIST

1. *Patient*

Sex	F
Age	24
Marital status	Married
Occupation	Receptionist.
Complaint	Frigidity.
What seems to bring patient now	Has been married ten months. Continuing frigidity after operation for stretching of hymenal orifice.

2. *Therapist*

Code	F
Sex	M

B. PSYCHIATRIC HISTORY AND DIAGNOSIS

Family history. Mother, very highly strung, had some sort of nervous illness two years ago, details not known. Sister suffers from (i) irregular periods and (ii) excessive hair.

Home atmosphere. Not unhappy, but (i) considerable struggle between patient and father, who 'always came off best'; and (ii) jealousy between the patient and her sister.

Menstrual and medical history. FMP at 12–13. Periods always irregular; natural rhythm seems to be 5–7/24–25, but sometimes may recur after ten days, sometimes not for two to three months. Discharge heavy; fairly severe pain on first day. Since puberty she has suffered from excessive hair on face and legs. Two years ago her 17-ketosteroid excretion was 15·4 mg./24 hours.

Present illness. Husband unable to rupture her hymen though as far as could be made out he had little difficulty with his erection. Six weeks after marriage, examination showed that she had an intact hymen with a small hole at one side. Uterus was anteverted and there was no other gynaecological abnormality. The hymenal orifice was stretched under general anaesthesia. Her husband was now able to penetrate, but she continued to have an extreme distaste for intercourse.

Diagnosis. Dr. S. L. Simpson, author of *Major Endocrine Disorders* (1959) gave his opinion on this patient as follows: (i) She suffers from a mild and familial form of adrenogenital syndrome, which is usually the result of pituitary-adrenal hyperfunction.

(The pilot's wife—continued)

(ii) Although the total 17-ketosteroid excretion lies towards the upper limit of what is regarded as normal, fractionation would probably reveal that certain androgenic hormones are being produced in excess. (iii) The *physiological* effect of these androgenic hormones in women is usually not to decrease libido but to increase it. (iv) Therefore, her frigidity is most probably psychogenic.

The final diagnosis is: Frigidity in a hysterical personality suffering from mild adrenogenital syndrome.

C. ALL KNOWN DISTURBANCES IN PATIENT'S LIFE

(a) *Inability to accept femininity*
Has always been a tomboy. Intense insistence on women's equality. Completely frigid. Gets no pleasure from intercourse. Suffers from vaginismus, but can just relax enough to let her husband penetrate. Allows husband intercourse two or three times a week 'which is more than most men get'. Can't bear the idea of having a baby.

(b) *Indications that she wants to be feminine but is unsure of her femininity*
Intense resentment against men who won't give up a place to her in the Tube.

D. AREAS OF PATIENT'S LIFE UNAFFECTED BY ABOVE DISTURBANCES

In spite of all above disturbances lives a normal, full, though superficial, social life; and seems, apart from sex, to have a surprisingly good relation with her husband.

E. MINIMUM PSYCHODYNAMIC HYPOTHESIS SUGGESTED TO EXPLAIN C

Intense jealousy of men; wish to be a man; feeling of inadequacy about her own femininity partly as a reaction to this, and partly as a reaction to the virilism which she shows.

F. EVIDENCE REQUIRED IN ASSESSMENT OF 'IDEAL' RESULT

(a) Ability to enjoy intercourse and achieve orgasm. Sex life satisfactory to both partners.
(b) Extensive evidence from her life of
    (i) reduction in her resentment against men and
    (ii) a complete acceptance of femininity.

G. THERAPEUTIC PLAN FORMULATED AT INITIAL ASSESSMENT

To try and get at the meaning of her resentment against men, through the transference if necessary, and to relate this to her frigidity.

H. SUMMARY OF COURSE OF THERAPY

This vivacious but relatively superficial girl revealed all her psychopathology at interview (session 1), but in session 2 spent her whole time chatting about trivialities. Just before the next session she rang up saying her husband had got into trouble and she wanted to put off treatment for the time being. She did not get in touch with the clinic for six months, after which she asked for further treatment through her gynaecologist. The need to block the therapeutic work, mainly by contradicting everything the (male) therapist said, crystallized at once, and continued in sessions 4, 5, and 6. Every session threatened to develop into an argument. The therapist allowed this to develop and interpreted it forcefully in session 6, suggesting that it expressed her need to reduce all men to impotence. He related this to her frigidity with her husband.

There was less evidence of strain in the next three sessions, but the argument again developed in session 10, and the patient successfully prevented effective interpretation. In the next session, however, she was somewhat depressed and much more cooperative, and expressed the feeling that *she* was failing. This led to the interpretation that she felt uncertain of her own femininity, to which she brought much confirmatory material—e.g. she said that the doctor had told her her 'male hormones were over-active'. This led in turn to the interpretation that in preventing her husband, or the therapist, from being a man with her she prevented herself from being a woman, and this was why she had felt that it was she who was failing. In session 14 she began behaving in a way which the therapist thought was flirtatious, but when he pointed this out she became extremely offended. Although the breach between patient and therapist was healed and the relation remained good to the end, not much further progress could be made.

WORK ON TERMINATION. There was one recorded interpretation about disappointment over termination, to which the patient agreed but added that she had never believed in this sort of treatment anyhow. One interpretation about anger was denied.

Total no. of sessions 19
Total time 12 months

The present work

I. CHANGES IN ALL DISTURBANCES LISTED UNDER C

Follow-up (1) 6 months (information from gynaecologist):

Patient extremely upset, feeling that she might be pregnant. Her period eventually arrived some 3 weeks late.

Follow-up (2) 1 year:

She was happier and more relaxed, but herself said that this was mainly because her husband wants intercourse less often. No other changes. Nevertheless she was very pleased at the therapist's continued interest in her.

J. SUMMARY OF CHANGES. PSYCHODYNAMIC ASSESSMENT OF RESULT

Essentially unchanged.

Score 0.

K. STATUS OF THE EVIDENCE

Unequivocal.

THE RAILWAY SOLICITOR

A. DETAILS OF PATIENT AND THERAPIST

1. *Patient*

Sex	M
Age	24
Marital status	Single
Occupation	Assistant to a solicitor for British Railways. Not yet qualified.
Complaint	Severe headaches, depression.
What seems to bring patient now	Referred by a psychiatrist who had been treating him for 15/12, since he did not seem to be improving.

2. *Therapist*

Code	G
Sex	M

B. PSYCHIATRIC HISTORY AND DIAGNOSIS

Family history. Father had an accident when the patient was 7 and was then an ailing man till his death when the patient was 20. Mother has suffered from depression since the father's death.

Home atmosphere. Happy on the whole.

Previous history. NAD.

Present illness. He dated the onset of his headaches fairly exactly, about 2½ years ago. They are frontal, bilateral, and spread upwards and round to the back of his head. There is evidence that they are not due to eyestrain—e.g. they tend to be relieved rather than exacerbated by studying. No other physical cause was found. Fifteen months ago he consulted a psychiatrist and was taken under psychotherapy and drug treatment. During this period he began to suffer from anxiety, tension, and depression, the last consisting mainly of a preoccupation with the feeling that he was losing his powers.

Physical examination. The referring psychiatrist wrote: 'NAD. BP 132/80.'

Diagnosis. Anxiety neurosis, psychogenic headache, and reactive depression.

C. ALL KNOWN DISTURBANCES IN PATIENT'S LIFE

(a) *Symptoms*

Headaches for 2½ years. Feelings of tension.

111

(The railway solicitor—continued)

(b) *Relations with women*

Extremely shy with girls. Still lives with his mother, on whom he appears to be rather dependent.

(c) *Relations with men, problems over achievement*

Intense competitiveness with older men at work, accompanied by anxiety. He failed final exam twice, yet has I.Q. of 140. He has recently been depressed about the feeling that he is failing in masculine achievement and losing his powers.

D. AREAS OF PATIENT'S LIFE UNAFFECTED BY ABOVE DISTURBANCES

Efficient worker who does not let his symptoms interfere overmuch with his professional life. Good relations with men of his own age. Apart from recent exam failure has always been above average in intellectual achievements.

E. MINIMUM PSYCHODYNAMIC HYPOTHESIS SUGGESTED TO EXPLAIN C

Intense anxieties about competition with men, especially sexual competition.

F. EVIDENCE REQUIRED IN ASSESSMENT OF 'IDEAL' RESULT

(a) Disappearance of headaches.
(b) Ability to form satisfactory relations with girls. Ability to leave home.
(c) Reduction in competitiveness and anxiety about it. Ability to fulfil his potentialities at work. No further depression.

G. THERAPEUTIC PLAN FORMULATED AT INITIAL ASSESSMENT

Stated explicitly after session 3: to interpret intense hostility, rivalry, and fear in his relation to the therapist, and to link this with his relation to his father.

H. SUMMARY OF COURSE OF THERAPY

This patient was referred because his previous therapist was getting into difficulties. The patient was one of the type that never responds markedly to interpretations, but works with them gradually. A way into his difficulties via the transference was provided almost at once, since the patient seemed very uneasy at talking about his sexual difficulties, and the therapist interpreted that he felt resentful at having to reveal to another man that he was

(The railway solicitor—continued)

inferior in sexual virility—with which the patient agreed. In the next 10 sessions this focus of Oedipal rivalry was thoroughly explored in relation to the therapist and the patient's father. The patient spoke of how he never mourned his father; and there were indications that he still had the phantasy that his father might come to life and punish him. In the second third of therapy the focus shifted to heterosexual anxieties—his need to control his mother in order to defend himself against his fear of her, and the consequent need to identify with strong men.

WORK ON TERMINATION. As termination approached, there was some anxiety and intensification of his headaches, which led the therapist to make interpretations about anger over termination. There was no marked response to these interpretations, the patient withdrew, and the transference remained basically uneasy.

Total no. of sessions 30
Total time   3 months

I. CHANGES IN ALL DISTURBANCES LISTED UNDER C

Follow-up (1) 2 months (the day before his final exam):

(*a*) *Symptoms*. Headaches much milder, but still occur occasionally.

(*b*) *Relations with women*. He still feels that if he takes a girl out other men will laugh at him.

(*c*) *Relations with men, problems over achievement*. Anxieties about men are certainly still present, though whether they are reduced or not is not clear. He now admits anxiety about his exam, which he never did before. Depressions still occur, but are much milder.

Follow-up (2) 1 year 10 months (letter from patient, who has moved away from London):

(a) 'My headaches too continue to lessen in frequency, but the improvement is very gradual. But perhaps the biggest improvement . . . is that . . . I have very seldom felt depressed.'
(b) 'The one thing which causes me most concern is my continued fear of criticism of any relations I may have with the opposite sex, and as a result such relations are kept to a minimum. I realize this fear is completely unjustified but I do not seem to be able to put it behind me.' He is living away from home.
(c) He says that he enjoys travelling around the country on

113

business. 'I find that I am much more confident whilst dealing with such business matters than I was two or three years ago.' He has passed his final exams.

Follow-up (3) 3 years 4 months (letter from patient):

(a) 'Whilst I still suffer occasionally from the same symptoms . . . they are now much milder, and I feel that my condition is still gradually improving. Indeed, I feel there isn't room for much improvement, as I feel "on top of the world" most of the time nowadays.'
(b) 'No doubt the main reason for this is that I shall be getting married [shortly].'
(c) 'You will also be pleased to know that I am making good progress in my career; I find that I am now much more confident in my work, and my salary has increased by some 75 per cent since . . . three years ago.'

Follow-up (4) 3 years 8 months (letter from patient):

(a) 'I assure you that I continue to feel very well.'
(b) 'In answer to your last question, I have been enjoying married life for six weeks now.'

J. SUMMARY OF CHANGES. PSYCHODYNAMIC ASSESSMENT OF RESULT

Marked reduction in symptoms, with inappropriate reactions to both sexes apparently replaced by appropriate reactions.

Provisional score: 3.

K. STATUS OF THE EVIDENCE

This is a case in which the *post, non propter* argument may be applied with some justification. All improvements seem to have begun to occur relatively long after termination, that in the relations with women probably not for over two years. Moreover, although the facts seem incontrovertible, it is necessary to be guarded in any assessment that is not the result of an actual interview. In particular, there is no information about the quality of his relation with his wife. The evidence is therefore regarded as unsatisfactory.

THE STORM LADY

A. DETAILS OF PATIENT AND THERAPIST

1. *Patient*

Sex	F
Age	23
Marital status	Married
Occupation	Secretary-receptionist.
Complaint	Lifelong fear of death, now particularly in thunderstorms.
What seems to bring patient now	She is 3 months pregnant and feels she needs help with this fear if she is to have a family.

2. *Therapist*

Code	B
Sex	M

B. PSYCHIATRIC HISTORY AND DIAGNOSIS

Family history. Very severe neurosis in the family. Details not given for reasons of discretion.

Home atmosphere. Considerable conflict in the home between members of the family. Patient an unruly child.

Menstrual history. FMP at 13. Regular 4–5/28. No pain.

Present illness. She has suffered from this fear of death as long as she can remember. It later became particularly attached to thunderstorms. There were two isolated instances of this, first at 10 and then at 17, and it finally reached its present form three years ago when she was 20. Since then the intensity has hardly fluctuated at all.

Diagnosis. Severe chronic phobic anxiety state with underlying depression.

C. ALL KNOWN DISTURBANCES IN PATIENT'S LIFE

1. Known at initial assessment:

(a) *Severe phobias*
'A terrible fear of death.' This is seldom out of her mind. It comes on particularly in thunderstorms, also when travelling, so badly that she either becomes paralysed with fright or else gets into a real panic (e.g. during one storm sat half-way up the stairs with

115

(The storm lady—continued)

her head in her hands and couldn't listen to anyone; during another, couldn't go near a window and had to turn her back so that she couldn't see the lightning; still imagined lightning long after the storm was over). Is in constant fear that a storm will occur whether there is likely to be one in reality or not. Her reaction is severe whatever the severity of the storm. This phobia spoils her whole life.

(b) *Frigidity*

Intercourse at first painful, then bearable, but she has never had an orgasm. Feels she is not a proper woman.

2. Which came to light during therapy:

(c) *Depressive manifestations*

Therapy revealed that the phobias hid a complex and severe disturbance, mainly depressive in character. Manifestations of this included an inability to believe that she could be a normal mother or give birth to a normal baby.

D. AREAS OF PATIENT'S LIFE UNAFFECTED BY ABOVE DISTURBANCES

She puts on a very good front; and, apart from her behaviour in storms, has lived an apparently normal life and held down a good job.

E. MINIMUM PSYCHODYNAMIC HYPOTHESIS SUGGESTED TO EXPLAIN C

Far too complex for any useful simple hypothesis to be made. At assessment the hypothesis was made that her fear of death and the storm represented aspects of primitive sexuality and this was why she was frigid. There was evidence for this from an interpretation in the initial interview.

F. EVIDENCE REQUIRED IN ASSESSMENT OF 'IDEAL' RESULT

(a) Disappearance of the phobias.
(b) Ability to enjoy sexual intercourse.
(c) Extensive reduction in depressive phantasies.

G. THERAPEUTIC PLAN FORMULATED AT INITIAL ASSESSMENT

In view of the many emotionally charged responses that she gave in the Rorschach test, the plan was:

    (i) to show her one Rorschach card per session and to interpret her associations to it, with the aim

(The storm lady—continued)

(a) of getting at 'deep' phantasy material quickly, and

(b) of avoiding transference by interposing the card between patient and therapist;

(ii) for therapy to last 10 sessions, one for each Rorschach card; and

(iii) to interpret the presumed sexual meaning of her phobias— dying means sexual intercourse and the storm means the primal scene.

H. SUMMARY OF COURSE OF THERAPY

At the initial interview (session 1) the therapist resolved a tense situation, in which the patient could not talk freely, by interpreting that *the storm represented powerful primitive natural forces which she was afraid would overwhelm her*. The patient relaxed and was able to talk with feeling about finding her father unconscious and 'looking like an ape' after an accident. The main interpretation in the next two sessions was that the storm represented her fear of submitting to the overwhelming male. In session 4 the patient broke down and *poured out a mass of guilt and shame about childhood masturbation*. She said her façade had been broken down, and the therapist suggested that *she felt as if she had submitted to rape by him*. She then said, *'If there were a storm now, I would not be afraid.'* In session 10 the card reminded her of the inside of bodies, a mass of pulp. The therapist suggested that she felt that her inside was horrible (like faeces) because of the bad feelings which she kept inside her, *and when the baby was born it would turn out to be something horrible for all the world to see.* She admitted that her fear was that the baby would be shapeless or deformed. In the next session *she was able to feel the baby as something nice.*

This remarkable improvement was followed by at least partial relapse. Her anxiety during one storm was more severe than ever before. There were 19 sessions in all before she had her baby, and little further progress seems to have been made. In the last session the therapist interpreted the storm as representing her feelings about her parents in intercourse and her repressed sexual feelings about her father. Her final response was to say that she supposed these were subconscious feelings but they seem 'so remote'.

WORK ON TERMINATION. There is one recorded interpretation concerned with the patient's feelings about having to manage on

(The storm lady—continued)

her own 'without enough good things inside her' during her confinement, to which the patient emphatically agreed.

No. of sessions   19
Total time   6 months

I. CHANGES IN ALL DISTURBANCES LISTED UNDER C

Follow-up, 3 months (after birth of baby):

(*a*) *Phobias.* Apparently as bad as ever. 'Although there are no storms the fear of them is constantly with me.'

(*b*) *Frigidity.* No information at three months. Improvement occurred, but only after further therapy.

(*c*) *Relation with baby.* Extremely anxious about attending to the baby (a healthy girl). Unable to play with it.

Subsequent events:

She was taken on for treatment again at once. Therapy became stormy and dramatic, the patient ringing up in a desperate state and having to have extra sessions. Therapy continued at one session per week for a further year. Although definite improvements were found at further follow-up, these are not considered relevant to the present study.

J. SUMMARY OF CHANGES. PSYCHODYNAMIC ASSESSMENT OF RESULT

All disturbances essentially unchanged. (Also failure to terminate.)

Score 0.

K. STATUS OF THE EVIDENCE

Complicated by the fact that the patient was taken on again at once, but fairly unequivocal.

THE STUDENT THIEF

A. DETAILS OF PATIENT AND THERAPIST

1. *Patient*

Sex	F
Age	20
Marital status	Single
Occupation	Student nurse.
Complaint	Two recent thefts of money from fellow nurses.
What seems to bring patient now	Sent for treatment by her matron.

2. *Therapist*

Code	F
Sex	M

B. PSYCHIATRIC HISTORY AND DIAGNOSIS

Family history. Mother seems to be obsessional. Maternal grandmother now in mental hospital.

Home atmosphere. Parents have quarrelled constantly and have always been on the point of separating. Marked conflict between patient and her mother, persisting to the present day. Mother depicted by patient as demanding, unkind, and jealous.

Previous history. Difficult and unruly child, 'a terror'. But was head girl at her grammar school and very well thought of by her headmistress.

Diagnosis. Pathological stealing. For discussion see E below.

C. ALL KNOWN DISTURBANCES IN PATIENT'S LIFE

(a) *Stealing*

(i) At the end of a period of great strain, in which in addition to working for an internal exam she had to give support to a friend who felt she could not face the same exam, she stole money from this friend and a week later from another friend. There was great trouble at the hospital and she eventually admitted both thefts.

(ii) She was also accused by the matron of a number of petty thefts which had been occurring at the hospital during the last two years, and of two new thefts which occurred during therapy. These she consistently denied. No one knows to this day whether she was in fact responsible for them or not.

119

The present work

(The student thief—continued)

(b) *Relation to fiancé*

She is in love with a young man doing his National Service, and they plan to get married; but owing to practical problems they cannot do so for several years. This relationship turned out during therapy to be strongly idealized and, in view of the ease with which it broke up, largely false.

(c) *Relation to parents*

There is a great deal of conflict between her and her mother, particularly over her fiancé, whom her mother does not like. Patient has not been home for a long time.

D. AREAS OF PATIENT'S LIFE UNAFFECTED BY ABOVE DISTURBANCES

None

E. MINIMUM PSYCHODYNAMIC HYPOTHESIS SUGGESTED TO EXPLAIN C

There was disagreement in the Workshop about the diagnosis. Balint was convinced that she was a case of pathological lying as well as stealing and that she was in fact responsible for the other thefts. Therapist, and others, less convinced of this.

Evidence at interview suggested, and that obtained during therapy confirmed, that her main conflict was over maternal deprivation; and that this resulted in a conflict over giving and receiving love, care, and attention. The stealing would then represent her right to have something for nothing, without having to be grateful for it.

F. EVIDENCE REQUIRED IN ASSESSMENT OF 'IDEAL' RESULT

(a) No further stealing (or lying).
(b) Evidence of real and satisfactory relationship to a man, without idealization.
(c) Improvement in patient's contribution to the strain between her and her mother. Ability to tolerate her mother's failings.

G. THERAPEUTIC PLAN FORMULATED AT INITIAL ASSESSMENT

To try and deal with the idealization; not to lay great emphasis on the lying and stealing; if she is a pathological liar, to share in her phantasy but to help her to distinguish it from reality.

H. SUMMARY OF COURSE OF THERAPY

At interview (session 1) and throughout therapy the therapist showed a marked bias of sympathy for the patient and a feeling that she was entirely sincere. The Workshop's opinion was that

(*The student thief—continued*)

he had quite possibly been completely taken in by her. When in session 1 it transpired that the stealing had occurred after a long period of looking after another girl, the therapist interpreted it as *expressing her need for something for herself in return*. This seemed to make sense to her.

In session 2 the patient said that her fiancé, Reg, had been posted abroad and would soon be leaving. She failed to come for the next appointment, and there was then a gap of six weeks in treatment, during which Reg left. The gap ended when the patient was sent back by her matron after another theft had occurred, for which this time she denied responsibility.

In session 4 the stealing was interpreted as an attempt to bring home to her parents how much she needed. This led to the information that when small she had been paralysed down one side, *and her mother seemed to expect her to be grateful for the special care that she had received*. Although the patient had been twice *sent* for treatment, she now herself asked if she could continue, saying that she could not face her exams without help.

During the whole of the therapy there was evidence of some disturbance in the transference—a sense of constraint in the sessions, with the patient often arriving late. The therapist tried tentatively to bring this into the open in sessions 3, 5, 7, and 8, without success. In session 9 she arrived forty minutes late without apology, and the therapist finally brought out her *resentment that he took it for granted that she could come when it suited him*, whereas in fact it was not easy for her. The therapist at once linked this with conflicts over giving and taking in her relations with both her fiancé and her mother—in particular suggesting that she had been made to feel guilty about having once taken her mother's care for granted. The patient clearly understood this and said, 'And so, of course, I never go home'.

Therapy was terminated after the patient's exams two sessions later, and the therapist wrote in the notes that he felt he and the patient had had a very moving experience together.

WORK ON TERMINATION. None recorded.

Total no. of sessions   11
Total time   4 months

I. CHANGES IN ALL DISTURBANCES LISTED UNDER C

Follow-up: None.

After a great deal of acting out over an interview with an

121

independent assessor, to which she finally failed to come, she refused even an interview with the therapist. The only information comes (i) from a letter written by the patient 4 weeks after termination, and (ii) indirectly, through the matron, who let us know fourteen months after termination that the patient had eventually married.

(*a*) *Stealing* (*and lying ?*). No information.

(*b*) *Relation to men.* The idealized relationship with her fiancé broke down very quickly, and before the end of therapy she was doubting her feelings for him and had been meeting a West Indian student. In her letter (1 month after termination) she said that Reg had finally broken with her by letter. Within a year or less she had married the West Indian. There is no information about the quality of this new relationship.

(*c*) *Relation to parents.* In her letter she wrote that she had seen her parents twice since termination and 'we are once more a family'.

J. SUMMARY OF CHANGES. PSYCHODYNAMIC ASSESSMENT OF RESULT

Though it is possible that this girl was considerably helped both in her relation with her parents and in her relation with men, the refusal of follow-up suggests a highly unsatisfactory result in which the patient may have had much to conceal. If she was a pathological liar this was not touched. Marrying a West Indian may well be the expression of emotional problems, or bring new ones.

Provisional score 0.

K. STATUS OF THE EVIDENCE

Very unsatisfactory.

THE STUDENT'S WIFE

A. DETAILS OF PATIENT AND THERAPIST

1. *Patient*

Sex	F
Age	27
Marital status	Married
Occupation	Secretary.
Complaint	Fear of falling and hurting herself. Sudden onset eleven months ago, just before her marriage.
What seems to bring patient now	She has been supporting her husband, who is a student. Her symptoms have now forced her to give up work.

2. *Therapist*

Code	G
Sex	M

B. PSYCHIATRIC HISTORY AND DIAGNOSIS

Family history. Mother used to have fainting attacks.

Home atmosphere. Parents quarrelled a certain amount. Father spent little time in the home.

Previous history. Very timid as a child. Went through a period of having to follow her mother everywhere for fear that something would happen to her. Very afraid of men. Enuretic till 10 or 11 —much conflict with her mother over this.

Menstrual history. FMP at 15½. Regular 3–4/24. Little pain.

Physical examination. Gynaecologically normal.

Diagnosis. Phobic anxiety state with obsessional features.

C. ALL KNOWN DISTURBANCES IN PATIENT'S LIFE

(a) *Anxiety*
(i) *Phobic anxiety.* Her first anxiety attack occurred two months before marriage. She was frightened she would faint while waiting for lunch. This was followed by several more, e.g. while taking dictation. Since marriage the attacks have been much worse, and she now has a constant fear that she will fall and hurt herself which is so bad that she has had to give up work. Unable to travel

alone. Afraid she may panic in the street and have to run, and cannot wear high-heeled shoes.

(ii) *Obsessional anxiety*. For many years she has had the feeling that unless she touched something or wore certain clothes something might happen to her mother.

(b) *Sexual difficulty*

Although she has been married nine months she is not interested in sex and has not yet had intercourse.

(c) Constant restless movements observed at interview, suggesting the possibility of agitated depression.

D. AREA OF PATIENT'S LIFE UNAFFECTED BY ABOVE DISTURBANCES

No certain evidence.

E. MINIMUM PSYCHODYNAMIC HYPOTHESIS SUGGESTED TO EXPLAIN C

The hypothesis given in the test report was: 'Main problem seems to be concerned with conflict about giving up immature relations —mothering and being mothered—in favour of a mature sexual relation of which she is very afraid. She is afraid that her marriage entails the loss of her mother's love and approval. The picture is not that of a depressive.' This hypothesis would explain:

    (i) the acute onset of symptoms near the time of her marriage,
    (ii) her frigidity,
    (iii) her marriage to a younger man whom she has to support. The fact that her husband may now become self-supporting and thus more mature may account for her recent increase in anxiety.

F. EVIDENCE REQUIRED IN ASSESSMENT OF 'IDEAL' RESULT

(a) Loss of all anxiety.
(b) Great increase in sexual freedom: allows intercourse, with orgasm and enjoyment.
(c) Loss of restlessness.

G. THERAPEUTIC PLAN FORMULATED AT INITIAL ASSESSMENT

None specifically stated. Length of therapy limited by patient's planned departure to the United States in three months.

H. SUMMARY OF COURSE OF THERAPY

In sessions 1–5 interpretations were made about the possible sexual meaning of her phobias (e.g. fear of being hurt sexually, including fear of being 'penetrated' by therapist's interpretations); guilt about having a better marriage than her mother; and envy of her husband, whom she had been looking after while he studied for his final exams. There was some apparent response to these interpretations, but at the end of the first two sessions the patient pressed for advice as if this was what she was really seeking. In session 6, however, there was a much clearer response when the therapist said that the restless movements reminded him of a little girl wanting to go to the toilet. The patient responded by remembering that her mother had accused her, when she was a child, of *going to the toilet in order to masturbate*. After this session the restless movements were much less noticeable. Further response to interpretation seems to have been superficial.

WORK ON TERMINATION. One interpretation recorded, in the last session, with doubtful response.

Total no. of sessions   9
Total time   2½ months

I. CHANGES IN ALL DISTURBANCES LISTED UNDER C

Follow-up (1) 1 year (report from psychiatrist in Philadelphia):

Patient complained of
(a) Anxiousness at work, fear of being shut in the office, fear of collapsing in the street, inability to travel, fear of shopping;

(b) Fear of and lack of interest in marital relations.

Patient taken on for treatment. Seen at first twice weekly; then, because of the severity of her phobic symptoms, three times weekly. Total: 25 sessions.

Patient changed jobs twice and moved house twice during therapy. She finally encouraged husband to move to New York, requesting referral for treatment there.

During therapy there was a marked lessening of phobic symptoms and an increase in the ability to work, but there also appeared noticeable depressive elements.

Follow-up (2) 3 years 1 month (letter from patient):

Therapist received a letter from patient, who has now returned to England, requesting referral for further treatment. Patient reports that after each of the three times that she moved to a new city her symptoms at first greatly improved, but that after a few months she relapsed. In New York she had further psychotherapy and drug treatment, but the effectiveness of this was limited by her impending return to England (just as her first therapy was limited by her departure to America). She now says she gets depressed, her fear of fainting is 'almost an obsession', and travelling alone 'is out of the question'.

No further information about the sexual problems or the restless movements.

J. PSYCHODYNAMIC ASSESSMENT OF RESULT

Essentially unchanged.

Score 0.

K. STATUS OF THE EVIDENCE

Although the patient has not been seen since termination, unequivocal.

THE SURGEON'S DAUGHTER

A. DETAILS OF PATIENT AND THERAPIST

1. *Patient*

Sex   F
Age   29
Marital status   Single
Occupation   Editorial assistant to a magazine.
Complaint   ⎫ She had been engaged to a man, Dick, for
What seems to bring ⎬ over a year, but had broken it off on
  patient now   ⎭ discovering that he was still going out
                   with another woman. Shortly after this
                   the patient discovered that she was
                   pregnant. Sought treatment ostensibly
                   because she didn't know what to do
                   about this.

2. *Therapist*

Code   C
Sex   M

B. PSYCHIATRIC HISTORY AND DIAGNOSIS

Family history, home atmosphere. Patient is the child of a broken home. She felt a lack of warmth and understanding in her home.

Previous history. An unhappy, nervous, and resentful child, inclined to get depressed. Enuretic till age 10. Has always lacked drive; has never been able to stand up for herself; and has always been subject to fits of depression—crying and waking up early in the morning—when she has felt she has not measured up to her ambitions. Had a brief attack of a phobia of going into the Underground in early 20s. She was not depressed when seen by us.

Diagnosis. Neurotic character disorder and recurrent reactive depression.

C. ALL KNOWN DISTURBANCES IN PATIENT'S LIFE

1. Known at initial assessment:

These were not at all clear at first and were only pieced together by inference from her story, and with the help of the projection test (ORT).

The conclusion was that she had covered up her 'bad' feelings (hatred and sexuality) all her life, and pretended that everything

127

was nice. The test indicated intense underlying resentment against her mother; and her history showed that she expressed no resentment against Dick in spite of the fact that he had made her pregnant and abandoned her for another woman. There was no material about the baby in the test or the interview, which suggested she was denying the reality of the experience of being pregnant and giving birth to a child.

2. Which came to light during therapy:

It became clear that she was largely unable to express resentment, or to stand up for herself and her rights. It also began to look as if this pregnancy had been partly engineered by her—since she had made no attempt to prevent Dick having intercourse with her without contraceptives—as a way of forcing Dick to marry her without having to ask directly.

D. AREAS OF PATIENT'S LIFE UNAFFECTED BY ABOVE DISTURBANCES

There was no evidence of strong dependence. She had done fairly well academically and at work.

E. MINIMUM PSYCHODYNAMIC HYPOTHESIS SUGGESTED TO EXPLAIN C

Mainly inability to tolerate her own anger. Also, perhaps, anxiety over rivalry with women, with consequent anxiety over fulfilling herself as a woman by having a baby.

F. EVIDENCE REQUIRED IN ASSESSMENT OF RESULT

(a) The ability to experience the fact of being pregnant, and to have a normal relationship with her baby.
(b) Evidence that she is able to express her resentment and to insist on her needs with men in a way that makes the relationship better rather than worse.
(c) Same as (b) with women.

G. THERAPEUTIC PLAN FORMULATED AT INITIAL ASSESSMENT

A full therapy should have three main aims, to enable her to accept
(a) that she is really about to have a baby;
(b) that men don't necessarily have to be spared her resentment; and
(c) that there is a possibility of peace and friendship with a woman.
It was felt that the therapist should concentrate on (a), but

also might be able to achieve (b) through use of the transference; (c) could probably not be touched.

H. SUMMARY OF COURSE OF THERAPY

The main focus of therapy was how she had to be 'nice' all the time for fear of spoiling her relations with people, and thus could not be angry or press her claims. This applied in particular to the difficult triangular relation between herself, her fiancé, and her rival, which was pointed out several times in sessions 1–6. In session 7 the therapist pointed out how nice she had to be in treatment for fear of being thrown out; and in sessions 8 and 9 how she could not be angry or press her claims over the anticipated termination. The patient clearly understood all these interpretations but did not see how anything could be done to change the situation. In sessions 13–15 the therapist made a determined attempt (in accordance with the original plan) to face the patient with her feelings about her baby, with little success. In session 16 the patient announced that she had decided to get married, and in this session she contradicted the therapist and admitted that she was angry with him, for the first time. In session 17 she said that she now felt freer to express herself with Dick, but she was still uncertain what to do about treatment. In session 18 she said that she had decided to try and manage on her own, and the therapist agreed.

WORK ON TERMINATION. Interpretations about termination had already been made in the middle of the therapy (as mentioned above) and were apparently not repeated at the end.

Total no. of sessions 18
Total time   10 weeks

I. CHANGES IN ALL DISTURBANCES LISTED UNDER C

Follow-up (1) 5 months:

Not very long after the end of treatment things came to a head between her and her rival, and she had a terrific row and slapped the rival's face. At first Dick was furious with her; but, after the birth of the baby (a boy), everything has been different and they are planning to get married. It is not easy to get an accurate idea of the quality of her relationship with Dick. During therapy she was able to push him around a bit, and she is probably the dominant partner.

129

(The surgeon's daughter—continued)

The relationship with the baby seems excellent—the therapist writes: 'At the end of treatment I had no idea of the motherliness she could bring to her baby, and now it is evident that she has a considerable supply.' In view of the lack of response to interpretations about her denial of her feelings for the baby, it seems as if these interpretations may have been ineffective but unnecessary.

Follow-up (2) 1 year (interview with independent assessor):

She is now married to Dick. She describes her whole life as steadily growing happier—'like a spring being unwound as the tension is relieved'. She goes out to work by day, while Dick studies and looks after the baby; and he goes out to work some evenings. Still not easy to get at the quality of their relationship. Baby seems flourishing.

She describes the row with her rival: one evening the anger had simply boiled up inside her; she had felt that if she didn't do something about it now it would be spoiling all the good work that Dr. C. had done; slapping her rival's face had been 'most satisfying'; she hadn't done such a thing since she was 10. Interviewer asks if she has been more able to express such feelings since then, and she answers that she is certainly able to make her comments more pungent than they used to be.

Follow-up (3) 2 years (interview with same independent assessor):

Patient has recently had a second baby, which died. What emerged was (a) that this baby was unwanted, and (b) that the pregnancy had had the desired effect of forcing Dick to get a job and support her. Much of the interview was taken up with her guilty feeling that she had engineered the pregnancy, and that the baby had died after serving its purpose. It looks, therefore, very much as though this was an exact repetition of the mechanism of getting what she wanted without actually asking for it, which had been expressed in the original pregnancy.

She said she had never had any difficulty over sex; and the present sexual relation with Dick seemed to be genuinely satisfactory.

SUMMARY OF CHANGES. PSYCHODYNAMIC ASSESSMENT OF RESULT

This second pregnancy is strong evidence that the original problem over demanding her rights was not really solved; and that the ability to fight with her rival was a temporary effect occasioned by her relation with the therapist. Nevertheless she has apparently been enabled by therapy to make a tolerably happy marriage, and this must therefore be regarded as a 'valuable false solution'.

Score 1.

K. STATUS OF THE EVIDENCE

This is an inferential assessment, but the evidence from the second pregnancy is too much of a coincidence to be ignored.

Tom

A. DETAILS OF PATIENT AND THERAPIST

1. *Patient*

Sex	M
Age	16
Marital status	Single
Occupation	Schoolboy
Complaint What seems to bring patient now	Physical symptoms and anxiety of acute onset, four weeks.

2. *Therapist*

Code	B
Sex	M

B. PSYCHIATRIC HISTORY AND DIAGNOSIS

Family history, circumstances, and atmosphere. Mother discovered to be suffering from PTb when patient was 3, spent most of the rest of her life in hospital, and died when patient was 7. Patient remembers very little about her. Father remarried about one year later. Father was impotent, though one boy was born of the second marriage. There were constant quarrels, and the stepmother left the father three years ago. Relation between patient and his stepmother has always been very good, and she has treated him as if he were her own son.

Previous history. He seems to have been quite normal in his childhood and adolescence.

Medical history. No serious illnesses. No Tb. Three years ago complained of spot in front of the left eye, diagnosed as juxtapapillary choroiditis, which resolved spontaneously.

Present illness. Sudden onset of symptoms in the street at a time when he was due (i) to go for interview for his first job the next day, and (ii) to take his GCE exam the next week. His stepmother had several times during the last three years discussed the possibility of his leaving his father and coming to live with her as soon as she could find a satisfactory place to live. After the beginning of his symptoms she suggested that he should come right away.

Physical examination. Full clinical and neurological examination in a casualty department revealed no abnormality except a blood

132

(*Tom—continued*)

pressure of 180/75, presumably the result of anxiety. (All physical examinations and investigations after termination were also negative.) Chest x-ray normal. Because of his eye symptoms he also visited an eye hospital, where the old juxta-papillary choroiditis was seen and he was told that no treatment was indicated.

Diagnosis. Severe anxiety-hysteria. (It should be added that the extreme severity of his symptoms and the somewhat bizarre nature of some of his complaints has later raised the question of whether he might be schizophrenic. Against this, he has always made excellent contact at interview, and has never shown the slightest sign of psychotic thought processes.)

C. ALL KNOWN DISTURBANCES IN PATIENT'S LIFE

(a) *Anxiety and psychosomatic symptoms*
(i) *Attacks of physical symptoms* (four weeks, intermittently). Can't see properly; feels he is falling; heaviness in chest, breathing difficulty; pain in left half of face; feels his arms have gone dead.
(ii) *Anxiety accompanying above attacks.* Feels he is going to die, that there is something seriously wrong with him physically, that he is going blind, etc.

(b) *Character problems, etc.*
Insufficient evidence.

D. AREAS OF PATIENT'S LIFE UNAFFECTED BY ABOVE DISTURBANCES
Insufficient evidence.

E. MINIMUM PSYCHODYNAMIC HYPOTHESIS SUGGESTED TO EXPLAIN C
Severe conflict between his wish to go to his stepmother and his loyalty to his father, presumably with underlying Oedipal anxieties. The precipitating cause of his symptoms was probably the fact that he was just about to get his first job, and would then be more independent and more in a position to leave his father.

F. EVIDENCE REQUIRED IN ASSESSMENT OF 'IDEAL' RESULT

(a) Ability to make up his mind finally whether to live with father or stepmother; complete loss of symptoms; no further substitute disability; no further breakdown.
(b) Ability to get on with both parents without anxiety whichever one he decides to live with. Regular work, with advancement according to his potentialities.

(*Tom—continued*)

(c) Ability to form satisfactory relationships with people of both sexes.

G. THERAPEUTIC PLAN FORMULATED AT INITIAL ASSESSMENT

To try and clarify his feelings about the present conflict, with emphasis on Oedipal problems.

H. SUMMARY OF COURSE OF THERAPY

At interview (session 1) this very pleasant young man spoke surprisingly freely for an adolescent, but made only a limited response to interpretations. The interpretation that perhaps his symptoms represented his punishment for wanting to leave his father and live with his stepmother resulted in nothing more than a long brooding silence.

The therapist stuck to the plan of interpreting Oedipal guilt mobilized by the family situation, but the patient took most of these interpretations as advice that he had got to make up his mind about whether to leave his father or not. There was no clear-cut response to interpretation at any time. The only transference interpretation was in session 3, that he wanted to show how ill he was so as to force the therapist to take a decision for him. The patient agreed with this, and said he couldn't carry on like this and must decide soon. In session 4 he reported that he had felt that the therapist had given him a sort of ultimatum—the more he avoided his decision the more ill he became—and as a result he had gone to stay with his stepmother, and his symptoms had improved. The therapist tried to get him to look at his feelings about this, but failed.

Another appointment was made, but the patient rang up saying that he felt much better and did not need to come.

WORK ON TERMINATION. Not relevant; patient broke off treatment.

Total no. of sessions 4
Total time 4 weeks

I. CHANGES IN ALL DISTURBANCES LISTED UNDER C

Follow-up (1) 3 months (report from another psychiatrist):

As soon as he decided to go and live with his stepmother all his symptoms and anxiety disappeared, only to return with equal force one month afterwards. He refused to return to the original therapist and was taken on as an out-patient at another hospital.

Follow-up (2) 3 years 3 months:

Spent one year as a voluntary patient in a mental hospital. Now has been out of hospital nearly two years. Still suffers from symptoms similar to those that he had originally, and in addition from claustrophobia, agoraphobia, and a partial spasm in one leg. He faces his disability with courage and has worked at the same job ever since his discharge from hospital. Now seeking further treatment at the Tavistock Clinic. Put on group waiting list.

J. SUMMARY OF CHANGES. PSYCHODYNAMIC ASSESSMENT OF RESULT

An attempted 'false solution' by relief of external stress, soon revealed as valueless.

Score 0.

K. STATUS OF THE EVIDENCE

Unequivocal.

THE UNSUCCESSFUL ACCOUNTANT

A. DETAILS OF PATIENT AND THERAPIST

1. *Patient*

Sex	M
Age	31
Marital status	Married
Occupation	A chartered accountant in private practice.
Complaint ⎱ What seems to bring ⎰ patient now	Patient has been unable to make a living in private practice. He has now decided to give up accountancy and has been trying unsuccessfully to get personnel work. Now asking for advice about what sort of job to take.

2. *Therapist*

Code	F
Sex	M

B. PSYCHIATRIC HISTORY AND DIAGNOSIS

Family history, home atmosphere. Father extremely domineering and moody. Sister neurotic.

Previous history. NAD

Diagnosis. Neurotic character disorder.

C. ALL KNOWN DISTURBANCES IN PATIENT'S LIFE

1. Known at initial assessment:

(a) *Difficulty over jobs*
 (i) Failure at accountancy.
 (ii) Decision to get personnel work, for which he is not qualified.
 (iii) Has been turned down at interview for about 20 jobs in the past two years.

2. Which came to light during therapy:

(b) *Character problems*

These were not clear at interview, but his projection test and subsequent therapy suggested severe difficulties over competitiveness, aggressiveness, and making real contact with people.

D. AREAS OF PATIENT'S LIFE UNAFFECTED BY ABOVE DISTURBANCES

He did fairly well academically, and became a chartered account-

136

ant. He has also married, though little is known about the quality of his relationship with his wife.

E. MINIMUM PSYCHODYNAMIC HYPOTHESIS SUGGESTED TO EXPLAIN C

It seems clear that his character problems in some way interfere with his getting jobs. Probably (i) his difficulty over competitiveness makes him choose jobs which are aiming either too high or too low (he said this during therapy); (ii) his wish for personnel work expresses his wish to solve problems in his relations with people, but he is unqualified and unsuited for this; and (iii) he antagonizes interviewers owing to his problem over competitiveness.

F. EVIDENCE REQUIRED IN ASSESSMENT OF 'IDEAL' RESULT

(a) (i) He should get a job which satisfies him, and should make progress in it, in accordance with his undoubted abilities.
(ii) There should be evidence that this has been due to altered behaviour at interview, and that this kind of pattern does not repeat itself in future.
(b) There should be evidence from his life for extensive reduction in problems of competitiveness and for improvement in the quality of his human relationships.

G. THERAPEUTIC PLAN FORMULATED AT INITIAL ASSESSMENT

Formulated after session 3: '[To] bring out competitiveness with men, to relate it to inability to get a job; to show him how he has tried to over-compensate [for] fear of competitiveness . . .; perhaps later the relation with father . . .; and ease some of the tension which is obviously responsible for his inability to impress interviewing boards.'

H. SUMMARY OF COURSE OF THERAPY

At interview he steadfastly refused to admit, in spite of sustained effort by the interviewer, that he had any difficulties; and said that he came simply for advice about what sort of job he should get, and that he would like to join a group 'in order to study the group leader's methods'. Nevertheless, he eventually said that the sort of job he would like was one in which he found out what workers' complaints really were. The interviewer interpreted that he really wanted to find out what his own complaints were. Although there

137

seemed to have been very little communication in this interview, the patient wrote saying that he had been considerably helped and would like another. In session 2 the theme was competitiveness. In sessions 3–6 the patient started to get uneasy as soon as he had run out of material that he had prepared, and the therapist reiterated that *some problem in his relation with men was appearing in the transference, and it was this same problem that made him uneasy at interviewing boards.* In session 6 after a period of tension and thought block, the patient interpreted this himself as being due to *homosexual feelings for the therapist.* In the next session he reported that he had got a job which made it difficult for him to have further treatment. Therapist and patient agreed on termination.

WORK ON TERMINATION. None recorded.

Total no. of sessions 7
Total time   6 weeks

I. CHANGES IN ALL DISTURBANCES LISTED UNDER C

Follow-up (1) 10 months:

(a) (i) Has completely given up the idea of personnel work. His job is with a commercial firm, at a much lower salary than that he would have attained if he had been successful in his profession, and with apparently few prospects of advancement; but it makes use of his qualification in accountancy. He seems perfectly contented with this state of affairs. (ii) Therapist could get no evidence that his getting this job was due to altered behaviour or feelings at interview—patient denied this. More likely due to the fact that this was a more realistic choice of job than before.

(b) No evidence of any significant change in any of the character problems.

Follow-up (2) 2 years:

(a) Little change from above situation, still quite contented. Has had some increase in salary—'about average'—and is expecting another. Has been given more responsibility. Is studying to get further qualifications, but plays down the possibility of advancement in his present job, which seems to be greater than he wants to make out.

(b) Still almost impossible to get much idea of the quality of his human relations.

J. SUMMARY OF CHANGES. PSYCHODYNAMIC ASSESSMENT OF RESULT

The psychodynamic change seems to be that he has largely abandoned competitiveness. The inappropriate reaction has thus been replaced by another inappropriate reaction. Nevertheless, his present position is more realistic than his attempt to get personnel work, and the result must be regarded as a 'valuable false solution'.

Score 1.

K. STATUS OF THE EVIDENCE

Inferential, but very clear.

VIOLET'S MOTHER

A. DETAILS OF PATIENT AND THERAPIST

1. *Patient*

Sex	F
Age	42
Marital status	Married
Occupation	Housewife
Complaint	⎫ A complex family problem with an acute
What seems to bring	⎬ exacerbation. Details not suitable for
patient now	⎭ publication.

2. *Therapist*

Code	F
Sex	M

B. DIAGNOSIS

Essentially a neurotic marital problem with repercussions on the whole family.

Items c to g are considered unsuitable for publication.

H. SUMMARY OF COURSE OF THERAPY

Early sessions all pursued the same pattern—the patient would try to get advice about the problems of other members of the family, and the therapist would have to make increasingly forceful interpretations about the patient's own problems and the part that they played in the family situation. This led gradually to partial insight (sessions 1–8). The situation at home then seemed to improve considerably, at which the therapist suggested termination.

WORK ON TERMINATION. During sessions 3, 4, and 5 the therapist had suggested that the patient was trying to get the help and support from him which she had not got from her husband, without definite response. Threat of termination, however, made the patient upset and tearful. Interpretations about the patient's anger and grief at losing the therapist's support were made in sessions 11–15, leading to the expression of open feelings on two occasions, but without resolution of the situation. The patient was transferred to long-term treatment.

Total no. of sessions 15
Total time 5 months

I. OUTCOME

After the initial improvement the family situation relapsed severely.

J. PSYCHODYNAMIC ASSESSMENT OF RESULT

Essentially unchanged or worse.

Score 0.

K. STATUS OF THE EVIDENCE

Equivocal. In a situation of this kind it is impossible to disentangle the contribution of the individual members of the family. Further follow-up was completely obscured by long-term treatment.

TABLE 6 SUMMARY OF THERAPEUTIC RESULTS

A. 'OEDIPAL' PROBLEMS IN MALE PATIENTS

Patient, Age		Disturbance		Change in disturbance	Follow-up	Score
Biologist 27	Women:	Poor erection; premature ejaculation.	Women:	Considerable improvement in potency, greater enjoyment of intercourse; improvement in relation with wife.	5 years	3
	Men:	Homosexual feelings expressed in compulsive phantasies.	Men:	Phantasies still present; intensity varies. Some homosexuality 'sublimated' in relation with boss.		
	Symptoms:	Severe eating phobia.	Symptoms:	Eating phobia completely disappeared.		
Neurasthenic's Husband 50+	Women:	Behaves as a slave to his wife. Attends to her sexual needs instead of his own.	Women:	Extensively able to assert himself with wife. After period of attending to his own sexual needs with her, has given up intercourse because she is seriously depressed.	3½ years	3
	Men:	Extremely self-depreciatory in relations with colleagues. Allows himself to be paid at far less than his true worth.	Men:	Has demanded and received increases of salary on a number of occasions. Has been given more responsibility.		
Railway Solicitor 24	Women:	Extremely shy with girls.	Women:	Now married. No information about his relation with his wife.	3½ years	3
	Men:	Intense, anxiety-laden	Men:	Much more confident at work.		

Case		Disturbance	Outcome	Follow-up	Score
		competitiveness with older men at work.			
	Symptoms:	Headaches and attacks of depression.	Symptoms: Headaches and depressions still present; much milder.	3 years	1
Civil Servant 22	Women:	Cannot make contact with girls.	Very little change. Relation with girls is still largely in phantasy.		
	Men:	Feels very angry if his boss criticizes his work.	Little change.		
	Symptoms:	Agoraphobia and eating phobia.	Phobias completely disappeared.		
Unsuccessful Accountant 31	Women:	None known.	—	2 years	1
	Men:	Intense anxiety-laden competitiveness leading to his being turned down at interviewing boards for jobs. Unable to get a job for 2 years.	Probably no change in underlying disturbance, but got a job below his potential during therapy, made normal progress in it, and has held it ever since.		
Tom 16	Women: ⎫ Men: ⎬	Severe conflict over leaving his father and going to live with his stepmother.	Women: ⎫ Men: ⎬ Left his father and went to live with his stepmother. Broke off treatment.	3¼ years	0
	Symptoms:	Intense anxiety attacks with physical symptoms.	Symptoms: Immediately cleared when he went to his stepmother. Returned in full force 1/12 later. Essentially unchanged ever since.		

Table 6—continued

Patient, Age		Disturbance	Change in disturbance	Follow-up	Score
Paranoid Engineer 28	Women:	Premature ejaculation.	No change.	Failure to terminate	0
	Men:	Psychotic preoccupation with rivalry, submissiveness/assertiveness, and homosexuality.	No change.		
Articled Accountant 22	Women:	No heterosexual feelings. Homosexual episode precipitated by a girl showing some interest in him.	No change.	2½ years	0
	Men:	Acute homosexual episode. Very afraid of his boss.	Homosexual feelings have receded but not entirely disappeared. Relation with boss ended in serious row. Relation with new boss possibly satisfactory (insufficient information).		
	Symptoms:	Obsessional fear of making small mistakes at work.	Symptoms: Still worried about making mistakes at work.		

B. 'OEDIPAL' PROBLEMS IN FEMALE PATIENTS

Patient, Age		Disturbance	Change in disturbance	Follow-up	Score
Falling Social Worker 27	Men:	Sexual relations short of intercourse with disreputable men; platonic relations with	Has largely given up relations with disreputable men. Has had several marriageable boy friends,	3 years	3

Case	Initial symptoms / relations	Outcome	Duration	Score
	marriageable men. Symptoms: Fear of falling. Feeling of unreality. Compulsive work.	but still suffers from sexual inhibitions. Symptoms: Fear of falling: still present but worries her less. Feeling of unreality: disappeared completely. Compulsive work: no longer works compulsively.	7 months (new course of treatment)	2
Girl with the Dreams 24	Men: Dissatisfied after intercourse. Women: Bad relations with older women. Symptoms: Frightening dreams. Panic attacks.	Men: No essential change. Women: Improved relations with women. Able to be a good mother herself. Symptoms: Dreams less frightening. Still has occasional panic attacks.	2 years (new course of treatment)	0
Draper's Assistant 21	Men: Non-consummation of marriage. Symptoms: Mild phobias, of little importance in her life.	Men: No essential change. Symptoms: Mild phobias disappeared, returned later.	1 year	0
Pilot's Wife 24	Men: Frigidity. Intense resentment against men. Very unsure of her own femininity.	Men: No change.		
Student's Wife 27	Men: Non-consummation of marriage. Symptoms: Severe agoraphobia. Has had to give up work.	Men: Probably no essential change. Symptoms: No change.	3 years	0

Table 6—continued

Patient, Age	Disturbance		Change in disturbance		Follow-up	Score
Violet's Mother 42	Complex family problem. Details not suitable for publication.		Severe relapse in problem after initial improvement.		Transfer to long-term treatment	0
	C. ESSENTIALLY DEPRESSIVE PROBLEMS; AND PROBLEMS EXPRESSED SIMILARLY TOWARDS PEOPLE OF EITHER SEX					
Lighterman 30	Anger:	Cannot be angry with mother. Has outbursts against his children.	Anger:	Has 'had it out' with his mother. Relation with children greatly improved.	1½ years	3
	Symptoms:	Whole life affected by compulsiveness. Severe anxiety attacks and confusional states.	Symptoms:	Compulsiveness extensively replaced by reparative drive. Anxiety attacks and confusional states now largely replaced by agoraphobia.		
Surgeon's Daughter 29	Inability to be angry or to insist on her rights. Has almost certainly unconsciously engineered a pregnancy in order to make her fiancé finally decide to marry her.		Slapped the face of her rival. Eventually married her fiancé. Marriage reasonably happy. Had another unwanted pregnancy which forced her husband, who had been studying, to support her.		2 years	1

Case	Initial state	Outcome	Follow-up	Score
Storm Lady 23	Symptoms: Severe storm phobia. Depressive phenomena: Inability to believe that she can be a normal mother or give birth to a normal child. Sex: Frigidity.	Symptoms: Essentially unchanged. Depressive phenomena: Essentially unchanged. Unable to play with her baby. Sex: Frigidity probably essentially unchanged.	Failure to terminate	0
Hypertensive Housewife 34	Depressive phenomena: Typical clinical picture of severe depression. Anger: Men: Uncontrollable outbursts. Strong tendency to have relations with disturbed men. Symptoms: Headaches.	Depressive phenomena: Immediate relapse after marked initial improvement. Finally admitted to a neurosis unit. Anger: No information. Men: No change. Symptoms: No information.	Failure to terminate	0
Student Thief 20	Symptoms: Stealing. Men: Highly idealized relation with fiancé. Parents: Has quarrelled with them.	Symptoms: No information about stealing. Men: Broke off relation with fiancé. Made what sounds like a doubtfully suitable marriage. Parents: Has made it up with them.	Refused follow-up	0
Clown 24	Social anxieties with a paranoid flavour. Cannot realize he is now a father.	Now no social anxieties, but this is apparently entirely dependent on his taking drugs. Feels he is a success as a father and that this is not dependent on his taking drugs. Later heard to be seeking treatment again, but details unknown.	1¾ years	–

Table 6—continued

Patient, Age	Disturbance	Change in disturbance	Follow-up	Score
Dog Lady 33	Symptoms: Severe dog phobia. Has to control everybody so that they are nice and kind to her. Relations with people: Terrified of any situation in which instinctual feelings may be aroused, particularly of group treatment.	Symptoms: No change. Relations with people: Her anxiety was sufficiently reduced for her to be able to stay in a group for $3\frac{1}{2}$ years. This is not regarded as a valid therapeutic aim for the purposes of the present study.	Transfer to long-term therapy	–

CHAPTER 7

Psychodynamic Assessment and its Bearing on the Validity of Brief Psychotherapy

It is of course true that, if a worker approaches data of any kind from a particular theoretical standpoint, he will tend to emphasize those aspects that fit in with his theory, perhaps to the exclusion of other aspects equally important. Very probably these patients might appear quite different through the eyes of other psychoanalysts, let alone through the eyes of psychotherapists of a completely different school.

It is also true that if these patients were taken under analysis their neuroses would all, almost certainly, prove to be highly over-determined, so that the dynamic hypotheses given here must be regarded as greatly over-simplified.

Nevertheless, it can be said that this kind of approach often gives an extraordinarily coherent and intelligible picture. Moreover, if an observer waits for sufficiently long after the end of therapy, enough will often happen to enable him to give a very clear account of the extent to which the patient has and has not really improved, and to give a dynamic interpretation of all the events that have occurred. The clearest example of this is the Biologist. The evidence may be set out as below:

1. *Main disturbances*:
(a) Eating phobia,
(b) Diminished potency,
(c) Compulsive phantasies with a clearly homosexual flavour.

2. *Dynamic hypothesis* (based partly on evidence obtained during therapy):
Guilt and anxiety about repressed homosexual impulses now returning to consciousness. According to a standard psycho-

149

analytic interpretation, this kind of homosexuality may well represent a sexualized submissiveness to another man as a defence against intense anxieties about rivalry.

3. *Course of therapy*:
Therapist focuses on passive homosexuality and anxiety about competitiveness with men. This leads to the recounting of a memory concerned with homosexuality and eating.

4. *Improvements during therapy*:
(a) Complete loss of eating phobia,
(b) Improved potency,
(c) Disappearance of compulsive phantasies.

5. *Follow-up* (8 months, 3 years, 5 years):
(a) No recurrence of eating phobia.
(b) Permanent improvement in potency and the relation with his wife.
(c) Compulsive phantasies return in full force at times of stress, and are still present now with diminished force.
(d) In keeping with the interpretation of part of his homosexuality as a defence against rivalry, a new problem emerges: difficulty over achievement. This is now satisfactorily solved by his getting a job as second-in-command to a man with whom he can express his submissiveness without any thought of engaging in rivalry.

A plausible and apparently complete account can now be given of what has happened to this man's repressed homosexuality:

1. Some has been brought into consciousness. The pressure has thus been in some way relieved, so that he can now express his heterosexuality more freely.
2. Some has been 'sublimated' in his relation with his new boss.
3. Some is still expressed in his compulsive phantasies.

This example is admittedly the most striking of all, but there are others only slightly less clear, for example:

1. The Surgeon's Daughter, in whom the pattern of getting what she wanted through an 'involuntary' pregnancy—which was what brought her to therapy—was exactly repeated one year after termination.

2. The Unsuccessful Accountant, who by his choice of job so clearly *avoided* his problem over competitiveness (for a full discussion of this see pp. 165–6).

3. The Articled Accountant, in whom a disturbance which was

not conspicuous—though present—at assessment, namely the tendency to deny his feelings and withdraw, finally became dominant and largely nullified his considerable initial improvements.

I am far from believing that psycho-analytic theory represents the ultimate on all human problems; but I do find it difficult to believe that the viewpoint expressed here, one-sided and incomplete though it may be, does not represent at least an aspect of the truth.

THE BEARING OF THIS WORK ON THE VALIDITY OF BRIEF PSYCHOTHERAPY

The validity of brief psychotherapy cannot be separated from the validity of psychotherapy in general. This question was extensively discussed in my previous paper (Malan, 1959) and it is worth repeating and extending this discussion here.

The evidence would come ideally from a 'crucial experiment'—the comparison of a treated and an untreated series of patients, both of which were selected in exactly the same way. Such a study is extremely difficult to provide and for the most part other workers have adopted various compromises, of a kind which are perfectly legitimate and correspond to those adopted—where necessary—in all other branches of science. Although it is true that, with one exception known to me, these studies are not without objection, it is also true that they have almost entirely failed to provide evidence favourable to psychotherapy.

In particular, the evidence that there is a high rate of improvement of some kind in untreated patients is quite overwhelming and simply has to be accepted. In face of this evidence psychotherapists can only take up the position that either their work is really no use, or else there is a difference between the changes that take place in treated and those that take place in untreated patients, which the methods of assessment used so far have failed to demonstrate. The development of a more satisfactory method of assessment is therefore of the highest priority. It is chiefly as a contribution to this problem that the present work claims attention, and hence ultimately—but not immediately—to the problem of the validity of psychotherapy. At the same time, it is obviously true that psychotherapists are likely to go on working on the assumption that what they do is of some value; and the present work offers evidence about ways of working, which—though it suffers from many obvious defects—is nevertheless worthy of some consideration.

151

The minimum conditions that a satisfactory study of the validity of psychotherapy must fulfil may be stated thus:

1. the provision of adequate 'controls';
2. criteria of assessment which are clearly stated, and which are truly related to the variable that they are designed to measure;
3. adequate follow-up.

Of these three conditions the first is the most difficult, and—as already stated—the various compromises that have been attempted offer a partial solution and are in themselves perfectly legitimate. In particular, separate studies, by different workers, on totally different types of patient must be accepted. It is in my view the second condition that has never really been solved; and it is because of this that the question of the validity of psychotherapy still remains open.

In fact it would be more accurate to say that the second condition has never been solved *for adults*. There is one study, on children, which fulfils not only this condition, but both of the others as well. The following quotation is from my 1959 paper:

'Teuber and Powers (1953) reported an experiment in which 325 "underprivileged" boys were given guidance and counselling over an average period of four years, in the hope of preventing delinquency. The counsellors include psycho-analysts and client-centred therapists, and for part of the time worked under a psycho-analytically trained supervisor. The boys were matched with a control group of 325 boys who received no counselling. At the end of the experiment the counsellors believed that they had substantially benefited two-thirds of the treated boys. The final result of the experiment was that ninety-six of the experimental boys made a total of 264 court appearances for delinquency, as against ninety-two of the control boys who made 218 court appearances.'

This study will remain for many years the envy of any worker in this field. From the present point of view, its main advantages are not merely the provision of exactly comparable controls, but the use of a method of assessment which as well as being objective and quantitative was undeniably related to the variable which it was designed to measure—namely antisocial behaviour. There are ways of interpreting this result to make it less unfavourable to psychotherapy—for instance it could be suggested that there was an additional factor at work in the treated boys, namely a tendency for treatment to increase 'acting out', which masked a genuine therapeutic effect—but the one fact that treatment did not keep these boys out of the courts, which must inevitably have been one of its major aims, is completely inescapable.

This study—on a type of patient that is notoriously difficult to treat—is of course not directly relevant to work with the usual population of adult neurotics. Its relevance lies in the dreadful warning it provides to workers in this whole field—the present study included—and which is admirably summed up by the authors themselves: that but for the controls this would have been published as yet another piece of successful work, and therefore the burden of proof is on anyone who claims results for a given form of therapy.

The important difficulty with the general population of neurotic adults is the absence of any simple objective measure of improvement resembling that available to workers with delinquent children. This is one of the reasons why there is no work with adults of a status in any way comparable with that of the above study. The nearest approach seems to be the study on client-centred therapy by Rogers and Dymond (op. cit. 1954). These authors took an immense amount of trouble and yet did not quite succeed in making their study free from objection. They attempted to solve the problem of controls by (i) dividing the twenty-nine patients to be treated into two roughly equal groups, one of which had treatment immediately and the other of which ('own controls') was asked to wait for an average period of sixty days, that is about eight and a half weeks or two months; and (ii) providing a group of 'normal' volunteers, who underwent the same series of tests without treatment. Eysenck (1960, p. 707) objects to (ii) in the following words:

'It is difficult to see what purpose the so-called normal control group serves. No one has, to our knowledge, advanced the hypothesis that a group of normal people not subjected to any kind of psychotherapeutic or other manipulation should change in the direction of greater integration and better mental health.'

The obvious fallacy in this criticism lies in the naïve view that there is a sharp distinction between 'neurotic' and 'normal'. Nevertheless the criticism does have some force, since the motivation for change in people who are not suffering from difficulties severe enough to make them seek treatment must inevitably be less high than in those who do seek treatment in fact. Rogers and Dymond by implication do recognize this. Eysenck's objection to

(i) is, I am afraid, more cogent. He states that his counter-hypothesis is that 'spontaneous remission occurs among patients to an extent which equals the alleged effects of therapy', and that one of the most important factors in this spontaneous remission is the passage of time. It is of course obvious that spontaneous improvements must take on the average much longer than two months to occur—otherwise most waiting lists for psychotherapy would rapidly dwindle away and disappear. Therefore (a) the period of waiting for the 'own controls' should clearly be at least the same as (b) the period of therapy, or even (c) the period of therapy plus follow-up. Since (a) was eight and a half weeks, while (b) was, on the average, thirty-three weeks, and (c) was thirty-three weeks plus six to twelve months, the 'own-control' series cannot be said to be of much value.

With regard to the methods of assessment used by these authors, it is very difficult to give a firm opinion. They used a variety of methods, doing their best to make each as quantifiable and objective as was feasible. There is, unfortunately, objection to all of them:

1. I am not convinced of the ability of patients to assess their own condition, nor of people to assess that of their friends; and therefore, while I accept the usefulness of the quantitative methods applied in the 'self-ideal correlation' and the Willoughby Emotional Maturity Scale, I do not think that these methods measure true psychodynamic improvement very accurately.

2. I very much respect the care taken over assessment by the TAT, particularly the fact that the judges did not know the order in which the tests had been given; but—as already discussed on p. 46—I am strongly of the opinion that assessment of change should be related to the patient's feelings and behaviour *away from the clinical situation*, and that changes in phantasy material are simply not enough.

3. The third method of assessment was the 'counsellor rating', in which the therapist himself was asked to rate the personal integration and life adjustment before and after therapy, and also to rate the overall outcome of therapy, both on a nine-point scale. In accordance with my view that it is only a clinician (though not necessarily the actual therapist) who can really rate changes in patients, I feel that this is the method potentially least open to objection. The difficulty here is that there is no information given about the criteria used, so that the judgements given cannot be verified by the reader. The one saving factor is that the authors

give a full account of the therapy and the changes that occurred in a single successful and a single unsuccessful case. The successful case ('Mrs. Oak', already mentioned—see p. 25) is extremely convincing; but this is only one (and probably one of the most successful) among the whole series of twenty-nine patients.

In summary: although these authors did find a 'significant' difference in the rate of improvement between the experimental and the control patients, (i) the two kinds of controls provided do not fulfil the conditions required; and (ii) it is impossible to know what this improvement means either in terms of psychodynamics or in terms of the patient's real happiness and adjustment.

The two other controlled studies on adults gave negative results. The first is that by Barron and Leary (1955), who compared the changes on the MMPI scale in 127 treated patients, and in 23 patients who during the course of routine clinic work had to wait without treatment for at least six months. The fact that the experimental and control series were selected in different ways has simply to be accepted. Treatment was either 'brief ego-oriented individual therapy on a once-a-week basis' (42 patients), or group therapy 'with emphasis on current interpersonal responses' (85 patients), with a minimum of three months' treatment in either case. Therapists were psychiatrists, psychologists, or social workers, all with more than three years' post-graduate teaching, and with a psychoanalytic orientation. The average lengths of time between the initial and final assessments were about eight months for the treated patients and about seven months for the controls. The results of this study were that both the treated and the untreated patients showed significant improvements in their MMPI scores, and that there was really no significant difference between them.

The authors do not make clear whether most of the experimental patients were still under treatment at the time of re-testing. If they were, then the study is based on the naïve view that patients show a steady improvement from the time that they are first taken into therapy. In fact, it is a universal experience that they tend to get dramatically 'better' in the very early stages—an improvement which is usually psychodynamically unsound—and in the next stage many of them get 'worse'. This kind of factor is not taken into account. It is, of course, easy to pick such holes in other people's work. It is much better simply to say that this was a sincere attempt to study the effects of psychotherapy with a control series, and that as far as it went it gave a negative result.

Brill and Beebe (1955), in an extensive study of problems re-

155

lating to psychiatric disability in the American armed forces, included a very brief account of a comparative follow-up study of those patients who had and those who had not had treatment. These authors attempted to correct their figures for the fact that the patients who had been given treatment were probably those with the best personalities in the first place, by matching patients in a treated and an untreated series according to (i) the (presumably geographical) 'area' in which the breakdown had taken place, (ii) the pre-service personality and impairment, and (iii) the severity of breakdown. Treatment was divided into: A—not more than rest and sedation; B—individual therapy; and C—hospital routine. 'The three matched treatment groups (A, B, and C) were then compared as to health at separation and condition at follow-up with essentially negative findings. It therefore appears doubtful that there was any difference in the effectiveness of the three gross types of treatment.' Here it must be remembered, however, that the authors specifically state that the facilities for treatment in the armed forces were very limited, and that individual psychotherapy should 'by no means be thought of as either intensive or prolonged'.

In summary, there are objections to all the controlled studies with adults that are known to me; but, though it cannot be said that the evidence against the validity of psychotherapy is very strong, the evidence in favour of it is negligible.

Failing controlled studies such as these—which are extremely difficult to carry out in a fully satisfactory way—important indirect evidence about the validity of psychotherapy could be obtained if it were possible to know the *natural history* of neuroses, in the same way as it is possible to know the natural history of physical illnesses. In fact, such studies as have been carried out all indicate that the rate of remission in patients who (though not necessarily entirely untreated) have had no specific psychotherapy, is very high.

Eysenck (1952, 1960) quotes two such studies. The first, by Landis (1938), is an extremely extensive study of the records of all neurotic patients admitted to the New York State Hospitals between 1917 and 1934. He found that 72 per cent were discharged 'recovered' or 'improved'. Landis himself explicitly states the limitations of such a study; and, for our point of view, I do not think it need be taken very seriously. *Of course* patients improve in hospital—it is the kind of life they lead afterwards that matters. And anyone who has worked in a mental hospital, and has had to

156

make out summaries for patients on discharge, ought to be able to attach to words like 'recovered' and 'improved' something of their true significance.

The second study, by Denker (1946), is of greater value. The following quotation is also from my 1959 paper:

'Denker studied 500 consecutive disability claims in the files of an insurance company, in which the patient had been out of work because of psychoneurosis for at least three months, and had received treatment from general practitioners only. The patients were followed up through their general practitioners for five to ten years. Criteria of "recovery" were (a) ability to carry on at work for at least five years, (b) complaint of at most very slight difficulties, and (c) successful social adjustments. The results were that 45 per cent of patients "recovered" after one year, and another 27 per cent after two years, making a total of 72 per cent once more.' (Further improvements occurred later, bringing the total up to 90 per cent after five years.)

A third study is also discussed in my 1959 paper:

'The most important of these [studies] is by Saslow and Peters (1956), in which the method of assessment was by means of the psycho-analytically based multiple five-point scale of Miles *et al.* (1951). . . . These authors studied 100 consecutive patients who had had consultations . . . and who fulfilled the following criteria:

1. They had been diagnosed by Saslow himself as suffering from a "behaviour disorder".
2. They had had no more than two interviews, for various purely routine reasons: e.g. lived too far away, refused treatment, were expected to be able to manage, were thought unlikely to respond, or were simply asked to return for drugs at times of stress.

Eighty-seven patients were located. Follow-up varied from $1\frac{1}{4}$ to $6\frac{3}{4}$ years—in 80 per cent it was over four years. The results were:

"Apparently recovered" to "Improved"	37 per cent
"Slightly improved" to "Worse"	63 per cent.'

A fourth study is by Wallace and Whyte (1959). These authors studied the changes in neurotic patients who had been on the waiting list for psychotherapy for three to seven years. They obtained useful information on 49 out of 76 patients. Criteria of improvement were based on symptoms and socio-economic

TABLE 7 DETAILS OF STUDIES OF ADULT OUT-PATIENTS

Reference	No. of patients	Treatment	Length of treatment	Criteria of improvement	Length of follow-up	Proportion 'recovered' to 'improved'
Maudsley Hospital (1931)	1,721	Eclectic psychotherapy, modification of environment.	More than 15 sessions.	Not stated.	Not stated. Presumably none systematic.	69%
Neustatter (1935)	50	Drugs, reassurance, suggestion, explanation, psycho-analytic interpretation.	Up to 9/12.	Based entirely on degree of improvement in symptoms.	Not stated. Presumably none systematic.	64%
Luff & Garrod (1935)	500	Re-education, explanation, deep analysis, suggestion, hypnosis, speech training, occupational therapy, etc.	50% under 20x 39% 20–60x 11% over 60x.	'Much improved': free from symptoms, normal lives, usefully employed, able to meet difficulties with self-confidence and without relapse. Information largely by letter only.	Yearly follow-up for at least 3 years.	55%
Yaskin (1936)	100	Suggestion, drugs, encouragement, some 'partial analysis'.	2/52 to 4½ years.	Not stated.	'Some cases were checked by follow-up enquiries.'	58%

Curran (1937)	83	No 'intensive' psychotherapy.	Only 25 patients attended more than 4x.	Based on symptoms and ability to work satisfactorily and comfortably.	1–3 years	61%
Carmichael & Masserman (1939)	100 (includes 19 psychotic and 1 epileptic)	Treatment of physical conditions, sedation, environmental re-adjustment, super-ficial psychotherapy; in 3 cases psycho-analysis.	37 patients only seen once, others up to 18/12.	Symptomatic and occupational.	1–30 months	51%
Ripley, Wolf & Wolff (1948)	690 (psycho-somatic)	Reassurance, support, expression of feelings, dream analysis, sodium amytal abreaction, etc.	Average 9 interviews.	'Symptomatic improvement': sustained diminution in symptoms and signs over a period of at least a year. 'Basic improvement': depended on the patient having encountered a major threat in his life situation and having met it in a more constructive way and without symptoms.	More than 1 year	16% symptomatically and basically improved. 34% symptomatically improved.

Table 7—continued

Reference	No. of patients	Treatment	Length of treatment	Criteria of improvement	Length of follow-up	Proportion 'recovered' to 'improved'
Rosenbaum, Friedlander & Kaplan (1956)	210	Analytically oriented, by residents.	Once a week for average of 9/12.	'Apparently recovered': no symptoms, marked improvement in social adjustment, no return of emotional disorder under severe stress. 'Much improved': essentially as above but transient exacerbation under stress. 'Improved': definite improvement in symptoms and in one or more areas of social adjustment. But total adjustment not as good as before illness.	Not stated. Presumably none systematic.	70%
Ellis (1957)	(a) 78	(a) Highly active analytically oriented psychotherapy.	At least 10 sessions.	None stated.	None	(a) 63%

						(b) 90%
(b) 78		(b) 'Rational therapy.'				
Wolpe (1958)	210 (total of 3 series)	Reciprocal inhibition.	65% of 88 in one series had fewer than 40 sessions.	(1) Knight's (1941) scale: based on symptoms, productiveness, sex, personal relations, and ability to handle stress. Symptomatic improvement a *sine qua non*. (2) Willoughby Personality Schedule.	'No systematic follow-up study'; 45/210 patients followed up 2–7 years.	89%

status. The overall result was that $32/49 = 65\cdot3$ per cent were judged to be 'recovered' or 'improved'. A study of the rates of improvement in patients according to the length of time on the waiting list indicated—in contradiction to Denker's study—that no further improvement occurred after the first three years.

As is well known, what Eysenck goes on to do is to review the corresponding figures for all major studies so far published of patients who have had specific psychotherapy of any kind. It turns out that the studies of psycho-analysis give an average improvement rate of 44 per cent (66 per cent if patients who did not complete treatment are excluded); while those of eclectic psychotherapy give one of 64 per cent; as against 72 per cent for the patients without specific psychotherapy in the studies of Landis and Denker.

The details of some of these studies mentioned by Eysenck, together with others not mentioned by him, are shown in *Table 7*. Only studies of adult out-patients, in which the majority of the therapy can be described as 'brief', are included.

Eysenck's (1952, 1960) conclusion from his published figures is well known: '[The data] show that roughly two-thirds of a group of neurotic patients will recover or improve to a marked extent within about two years of the onset of their illness, whether they are treated by means of psychotherapy or not.' The question is, is this conclusion justified?

It seems to me first of all that if the criteria used are the relatively coarse ones of (i) improvement in presenting symptoms and (ii) ability to work, then the evidence does really suggest that about two-thirds of neuroses are self-limiting, and that specific psychotherapy shows no *ultimate* advantage over such measures as rest and sedation—whether or not it *accelerates* recovery does not appear from the evidence available.

But what happens if the assessment criteria are more exacting than this? The seemingly most cogent argument used by the defenders of psychotherapy (including myself) is that dynamically oriented therapists use far stricter criteria. A consequence might well be that those studies in which such criteria were used would show a lower rate of improvement—although an obscuring factor will be the presumably different effectiveness of different kinds of treatment.

1. With regard to *untreated patients* there is perhaps some evidence for this in that the study by Saslow and Peters, making use of the psycho-analytically based 5 × 5 point scale of Miles *et al.* (1951) (which surveys work, personal relations, marital adjustment,

162

sexual adjustment, and insight), gave an improvement rate of only 37 per cent. This may be compared with the study by Wallace and Whyte (1959), giving a rate of improvement of 65 per cent, in which the criteria were much less exacting:

'1. Recovered: these were symptom-free and in full employment, and had suffered no loss in socio-economic status.

2. Improved: these were troubled only by residual symptoms, were in full employment, and had suffered no loss in socio-economic status.'

2. With regard to *brief psychotherapy* there is only one study that supports this idea, namely the psychosomatic study by Ripley *et al.* (1948), in which only 16 per cent of patients showed both 'symptomatic' and 'basic' improvement. There can be no question that these authors' definition of 'basic' improvement is highly exacting, and probably lies far closer to what I mean by 'true resolution' than improvements accepted by many other authors—depending as it does on the patients 'having encountered a major threat in their life situation, and having . . . [met] it in a more constructive way and without symptoms'. On the other hand, the somatic factor in these patients may make them more difficult to treat. The other studies in which the criteria were at least fairly strict give improvement rates which were either about average or above average: Luff and Garrod (1935) specify that the 'much improved' patients must have been able to 'meet new difficulties with self-confidence and without relapse', and these authors give an improvement rate of 55 per cent; Rosenbaum *et al.* (1956) also take into account the ability to withstand 'severe stress' and give an improvement rate of 70 per cent; while Wolpe (1958), using Knight's (1941) psycho-analytically based scale surveying symptoms, productiveness, sex, personal relations, and ability to handle stress, gives an improvement rate of 89 per cent. Moreover, in Wolpe's study a number of detailed case histories suggest that at least sometimes the kind of improvement effected is in no way different from those which occurred in our own work (e.g. see Wolpe, p. 127, a girl who showed a great improvement in her personal relations after discovering the ability to assert herself —cf. the Neurasthenic's Husband, p. 99 above).

3. As far as some of the studies of *psycho-analysis* are concerned, it is clear that the criteria—at least for 'recovered' and 'much improved'—are far more exacting than those used in most of the studies of eclectic psychotherapy, and it is therefore perhaps not surprising that the improvement rates should be lower.

This may be illustrated by quotations (a) from Fenichel (1930, my translation):

'We have been as strict as possible with the category "recovered". We only include those cases whose outcome is established not merely by disappearance of symptoms, but also by changes in the condition which are completely understandable analytically, and if possible by follow-up as well. Because of this strictness one can for all practical purposes include most of the "much improved" cases in the category "recovered". "Improved" cases include those which have either proved refractory in one way or another, or which must be considered only partial results on other grounds, or which must be dismissed as "transference cures" which are analytically doubtful.'

And (b) from Alexander (1937):

['Apparently cured' and 'much improved' are used 'most conservatively'.] 'They do not refer to patients who were merely freed from their symptoms, but a substantial improvement of the pathological condition was required. We call patients "much improved" who are no longer seriously handicapped by the remnants of their original ailment; from a practical point of view they are cured. "Apparently cured" patients did not show even such remnants of the original ailment. Patients whom we call "improved" we consider therapeutically unsuccessful because, though improved, they are still handicapped by their ailment.'

Fenichel gave an improvement rate of 39 per cent and Alexander of 50 per cent, which taken together lie well below the average for other forms of psychotherapy.

One thing only can be said: that the figures published by different workers are in no way comparable, and it is impossible to know what they really mean.

Although this is so, it nevertheless remains true that there is not the slightest indication from the published figures that psychotherapy has any value at all. If psychotherapy really is of value—and as a psychotherapist I find difficulty in believing that it is not—then how can this paradox be resolved?

It seems to me that a possible fallacy in all the figures so far published (except perhaps those of Ripley *et al.* and those from psycho-analysis) may still lie in the methods of assessment used. It is possible that two *qualitatively different* types of 'improvement'

164

may well hitherto have been classed together, namely (i) the 'true resolution', and (ii) the 'false solution', which is often of the utmost value in practice, yet remains dynamically suspect.

This latter kind of change is best illustrated by a detailed study of a single case from our own series, the Unsuccessful Accountant:

Here the 'presenting symptom' was an inability to be successful at his present job as an accountant in private practice and an inability to get another. This inability had been put to the test in twenty to thirty interviews during the previous two years. The patient was married, and his relation with his wife and his social relations in general did not contain any very obvious stress.

The bald statement of this patient's 'improvement' at five-year follow-up[1] is as follows:

> He got a job during therapy. He is still working for the same firm, with increased responsibility, and he has obtained rises in salary totalling about £1,400 a year.

It seems to me that the majority of the authors whose work is summarized in *Table 1* could not help assessing this patient as 'apparently cured'. But this assessment depends entirely on the lack of sharpness of the assessor's psychodynamic eye. The psychodynamic evidence will now be presented:

1. Therapy revealed in this man clear signs of an intense anxiety about competition and a difficulty in his relation with men in general, which might well account for his failure in his chosen job and his difficulty in being accepted for a new one.

2. In his relation with male members of the clinic this difficulty was manifested in that (a) he seriously antagonized the psychologist, and (b) in his therapeutic sessions he repeatedly could find nothing to say, and suffered from severe tension and moments of thought block.

3. The job that he got during treatment was a safe one, in which the element of competition was far smaller than in his previously chosen career.

4. Since therapy he has attempted to take a further examination. In spite of his high intelligence he failed in a subject in which he had specialized knowledge, and when he took the same subject again he got so anxious that he walked out.

5. He admits that he still feels very tense—he is managing in spite of this, but under considerable strain.

[1] This is a later follow-up which has become available since the Assessment and Therapy Form was completed.

165

6. In the presence of the therapist at follow-up he again suffered from great tension and moments of thought block.

It is quite clear that this man, who indeed has done very well in the externals of life, suffers from almost as much anxiety about competition, achievement, and his relation with men in general as he ever did. In other words, the underlying pathological process is essentially unchanged.

This conclusion is not based on any very abstruse psychodynamic theory, and when the facts are presented they seem to me very compelling; but it may take a knowledge of psychodynamic theory to see them in the first place. Yet if they are not seen the patient will probably be classed as 'apparently cured'; whereas if they are seen the patient must inevitably be judged dynamically to be 'essentially unchanged'.

The point that this case illustrates is that, since an independent observer has no means of knowing the degree of psychodynamic perceptiveness shown by any of the authors whose work has been described above, he has no means of knowing the proportion of *dynamically* improved patients in any of the series studied. This applies even to the apparently rigorous scales of assessment which survey different areas of the patient's life such as that of Knight, used by Wolpe. This scale might be applied to the above patient thus:

	Position before therapy	Change since therapy
1. Symptoms	None	No change
2. Productiveness	Severely impaired	Marked improvement
3. Sex	Apparently undisturbed	No change
4. Personal relations	Apparently undisturbed	No change
5. Ability to handle stress	Apparently undisturbed	No change

The psychodynamic approach, on the other hand, which makes as its starting-point an attempt to explain the patient's presenting complaint, enables one to see that in fact: (i) personal relations were severely disturbed; (ii) this disturbance was not altered by therapy; and (iii) the increase in productiveness was bought at the expense of a withdrawal from the anxiety-provoking situation. Which authors would see this and which would not? One simply cannot tell. This is why (a) the introduction of the psychodynamic hypothesis, and (b) the publication of the evidence on which the hypothesis and the final assessment are based, are so essential in studying the results of any form of psychotherapy. As far as I know, there is no study other than our own in which both these principles are recognized.

This distinction between 'resolution' and 'false solution' introduces a qualitative difference between results which does not appear in the published figures. There is, similarly, a quantitative difference which is most likely to appear in a comparison of the results of brief psychotherapy with those of psycho-analysis. This is best illustrated by a psycho-analytic case of Schjelderup's (1955). The patient was a woman of 42 who had suffered from compulsive doubt affecting almost every thought for twenty-one years, accompanied by a feeling of 'dislike' which destroyed all the pleasure in life. Obviously, if this woman could lose these two symptoms and find her whole life becoming more harmonious, she might well be classed as 'apparently cured', whether the assessor were dynamically oriented or not. But suppose—as happened in fact—that, *in addition to* these two changes, she not only discovered for the first time in her life the ability to express tenderness, but also found that the whole world had become more real for her, how is she to be assessed now? There is no category higher than 'apparently cured' to give her.

In my 1959 paper I concluded:

'. . . that studies of treated and untreated patients using crude rating scales are of little further value; and that a far greater contribution can be made by qualitative studies of even only a few patients with a method of assessment based on psycho-dynamics.'

The present work is an attempt to begin implementing the aspirations expressed in this paragraph.

Although the provision of a control series in the present work would probably not have been impossible, it would have been extremely difficult. One of the main difficulties was this: according to our original ideas, the most suitable kind of patient for brief psychotherapy was one who had a particular reason to be treated *now*. In fact, at least ten of the twenty-one patients studied fell into this category. It would have been ethically difficult to refuse such patients treatment; yet if we treated all of them we would not have been able to include them in the experimental series because there would have been no corresponding controls. In other words, there was an intrinsic difficulty in providing controls for the very type of patient that we wanted to study. Moreover, we had difficulty enough in finding such patients who were also suitable in other ways, without having to reject half of them automatically.

Although, therefore, we failed to overcome the problem of controls, we may perhaps claim to have overcome some of the other disadvantages of most of the work reported in the literature. First, we present in full the case histories of all the patients treated, so that independent observers can apply their own methods of assessment to them. Second, I think the method of assessment itself is an advance on those used previously. And third, the care and attention to detail over follow-up are (to my knowledge) unparalleled elsewhere, even in the excellent study by Schjelderup already mentioned. In other words, the way in which our work claims to go beyond previous work is that it provides a *basis* for *true comparison* of results, though it does not as yet provide the actual comparison. The question of the validity of brief psychotherapy, and of psychotherapy in general, can be settled only by a similar and extensive study of the changes that take place in patients under different conditions, but especially without treatment. This is a major undertaking and an entirely different project.

CHAPTER 8

The Therapeutic Results and the Problem of relating them to other Factors

In view of the evidence presented above, it is quite possible to maintain that the changes that took place in the present series of patients were not a consequence of therapy at all. Although, strictly speaking—without a study of 'controls'—this argument is unanswerable, it can be somewhat weakened by showing a coincidence in time between therapy and the onset of improvement. This applies particularly to *brief* psychotherapy in *chronic* cases. The clearest example is the Biologist, who had suffered from his eating phobia for three and a half years and who lost it permanently during a course of treatment lasting only five weeks. In two other cases: the Neurasthenic's Husband, with whom the symptoms had lasted for at least fifteen years and therapy lasted for five months; and the Falling Social Worker, with whom the corresponding periods were ten years and four months respectively; a graph of the severity of disturbances against time would show a sudden change in direction towards 'improvement' coinciding with a point soon after the beginning of therapy, with most of the improvement maintained permanently thereafter. In fact, of the nine patients judged to have shown worth-while 'improvement', in only one (the Railway Solicitor) did the improvements fail to begin during therapy or shortly afterwards.

In consequence, although the majority of the following studies on these patients are based on *correlations* and therefore include no assumption whatever about causality, the implicit assumption is always present that the outcome in each case is at least partly due to the therapeutic process. But it must always be remembered that there is no evidence at all to suggest the extent to which any change may have occurred as a result of processes quite independent of therapy.

169

The present work

This leads at once to the question of the *quality* of the improvements. It must first be recognized that even the best of these therapeutic results (with the possible exception of that in the Railway Solicitor) are very incomplete. Thus the Neurasthenic's Husband is left with a highly unsatisfactory relation with his wife, though admittedly this is not entirely under his own control; the Biologist still expresses homosexual tendencies in his compulsive phantasies; the Falling Social Worker still seems to suffer from sexual inhibitions; and the Lighterman's position, even if his phobias have disappeared, is almost certainly unstable. If our results are compared with the best of those reported from full-scale analysis (in particular those of Schjelderup, 1936 and 1955), they can be clearly seen to be inferior. This means that the score of 3 for outcome, the highest among our patients, is far from the highest possible. On this scale Schjelderup's patient mentioned on p. 167 above would probably score at least 6. On the other hand, it is my opinion that the present results do stand comparison with some of the best of those from long-term run-of-the-mill psychotherapy. Here it must be emphasized, of course, that our series of patients was very highly selected.

Our work provides almost conclusive evidence against the conservative view already quoted, that the results of brief psychotherapy are only *temporary* (Lewis, quoted by Gutheil, 1945). A continuous follow-up of three to five years cannot be dismissed lightly. In fact, I have myself been surprised at the low relapse rate among those patients who were still maintaining improvements a few months after therapy. If the special problem of the Draper's Assistant (who was thought to have improved but in fact was distorting the truth) is left out of account, the only examples of this are the Surgeon's Daughter and the Articled Accountant.

The other conservative view, that the results are only *palliative* (Rado, quoted by Gutheil, 1945), can only be answered by saying that such changes as the ability of the Neurasthenic's Husband to assert himself, or the reduction in the 'splitting' of men in the Falling Social Worker, or the replacement of the compulsive by the reparative drive in the Lighterman, consist of improvement not merely in 'symptoms' but in long-standing neurotic behaviour patterns, of a kind which longer and more intensive forms of therapy aim to achieve.

The therapeutic results are very heterogeneous, and thus suggest hardly any generalizations at all. But this heterogeneity is itself a generalization, confirming the radical conclusions explicitly stated by such authors as Pumpian-Mindlin (op. cit. 1953)—that good

170

results can be obtained (i) in a wide variety of cases and (ii) not only in cases in which the psychopathology is relatively mild and the symptoms are relatively recent.

In other words, our results may well contradict Hypothesis A, which is concerned with selection criteria—the next main subject to be discussed.

THE SCORING OF THE RESULTS FOR STATISTICAL PURPOSES

The distribution of scores on the four-point scale for outcome is shown in *Table 8*. Obviously, the scoring is non-parametric—

TABLE 8 DISTRIBUTION OF SCORES FOR OUTCOME

Patient	*Therapist*	*Score for outcome*
Biologist	B	3
Lighterman	F	3
Neurasthenic's Husband	E	3
Falling Social Worker	G	3
Railway Solicitor	G	3
Girl with the Dreams	A	2
Civil Servant	A	1
Surgeon's Daughter	C	1
Unsuccessful Accountant	F	1
Draper's Assistant	A	0
Storm Lady	B	0
Tom	B	0
Hypertensive Housewife	D	0
Pilot's Wife	F	0
Student Thief	F	0
Paranoid Engineer	F	0
Violet's Mother	F	0
Articled Accountant	F	0
Student's Wife	G	0
Clown	B	–
Dog Lady	F	–

Note: Though the patients are arranged in groups in descending order of favourable outcome, the order within each group is based upon factors irrelevant to outcome.

171

nothing more is implied than that a result which scores 3 is 'better' than one which scores 2 and so on. I consider that the scoring of most results is reasonably accurate. I do not believe, for instance, that any dynamically oriented observer could possibly regard the result in the Civil Servant as in any way comparable with that in the Falling Social Worker, in spite of the fact that the phobic symptom in the Falling Social Worker remains, whereas that in the Civil Servant has completely disappeared. Similar considerations apply to any pair of therapies whose scores differ by more than one point. There are, however, some doubts about the following:

Patient	Score	Reason for doubt
Railway Solicitor	3	No information about the quality of the relation with his wife. If this is satisfactory, perhaps the score should be 4; if unsatisfactory, perhaps 2. Improvement occurred so late after termination that perhaps it had nothing at all to do with therapy.
Lighterman	3	Very difficult to assess because of the replacement of anxiety attacks by phobias, the meaning of which is not clear.
Girl with the Dreams	2	A highly intuitive assessment. Perhaps she should score 1.
Student Thief	0	Insufficient information owing to failure of follow-up. There may have been important improvements. The assessment is intuitive.

The scores for outcome will be regarded as inviolable from now on.

THE RELATION BETWEEN THE CLINICAL AND THE STATISTICAL APPROACHES

The essential advantages of the *clinical* approach over the purely statistical are that (i) it can provide evidence on cause and effect (e.g. if a particular interpretation was immediately followed by a given improvement); (ii) it can give different weights to the evidence supplied by different individual cases and, above all, can exclude (a) those cases that fit in with a given hypothesis but for the wrong reasons, and (b) those that fail to fit in with a hypothesis but probably do so only because some other more powerful factor was at work. The disadvantage of this is of course that the argument can so easily become circular. One can always find a justification for explaining away any 'exception' if one tries hard enough.

The advantages of the purely *statistical* approach over the clinical are that (i) it combines all the evidence into a single quantitative statement; (ii) it can free itself from any danger of circular argument; and (iii) it can give a clear figure for the probability of obtaining a given result by chance alone. Yet there are serious accompanying dangers: (a) the figures may give an entirely false appearance of exactness, (b) there may be obvious clinical fallacies which have been overlooked, and (c) when the numbers are small, one or two 'exceptions'—which can easily be explained clinically—may completely spoil a correlation which is nevertheless quite real. Yet if one starts omitting patients on various excuses one can obviously reach any conclusion whatsoever.

It seems to me that the solution to this dilemma is, if possible, to use both approaches successively on the same data.

There are two obvious difficulties in applying the statistical approach to the present data: (i) Judgements are mostly retrospective. The only way to overcome this is to set down all the evidence on which the judgements are based. (ii) It is necessary to avoid the fallacy already mentioned (pp. 16–17) of taking figures for the 'significance' of individual correlations at their face value, when in fact many different correlations have been studied. For this reason the word 'significance' is used only for its convenience and is always put in inverted commas. A figure for the 'significance level' or the 'probability' (always for the two-tailed[1] test throughout the following studies) has to be given, since otherwise correlation coefficients of intermediate value are meaningless. I wish to state once and for all that I do not take these figures literally. And finally, the whole theme of this study will be, in the end, that the

---

[1] In the two-tailed test a positive and a negative correlation are regarded as possible, and the probability is calculated that the correlation coefficient will be *numerically* equal to or greater than a certain minimum value, whether positive or negative. In the one-tailed test only positive or only negative correlations are considered. The probability calculated in the two-tailed test is twice that in the one-tailed. The two-tailed is thus the more conservative; and it must be used when no firm prediction has been made in advance of whether the correlation will be positive or negative.

cogency of any conclusions drawn from the data is not derived from any individual correlation, but from the evidence regarded as a whole.

STATISTICAL METHODS USED

During several years of studying these data, I have learned much not merely about the relation between the clinical and the statistical approaches but, simply, about statistics. I have learned the hard way and made many mistakes. I should here like to acknowledge once more with grateful thanks the constant patience shown by Dr. A. R. Jonckheere in advising me on these problems.

The particular correlation coefficient used throughout the work is Kendall's τ (tau) (Kendall, 1955), which may be described thus:

Let us suppose that a series of individuals can be assigned a rank order (without ties) on each of two variables, A and B. It is now possible to select at random any pair of individuals and to record whether or not the member of the pair which is the higher in the rank order for A is also the higher in the rank order for B. τ_a represents the proportion of the total possible combinations which lie in the same order for the two variables, minus the proportion which lie in the opposite order. Since, if N is the total number of individuals, the total number of possible pairs is $\frac{1}{2}N(N-1)$, τ_a is given by the formula:

$$\tau_a = \frac{\text{(No. in same order)} - \text{(No. in opposite order)}}{\frac{1}{2}N(N-1)}$$

or

$$\frac{S}{\frac{1}{2}N(N-1)}$$

τ_a has the convenient property, shared by certain other correlation coefficients, of varying between $+1$ for perfect positive correlation, through 0 for no correlation, to -1 for perfect negative correlation.

When there are ties—to any extent—in either or both rank orders, τ can still be used, though no score is obtained from pairs of individuals which tie on one or other of the rankings. In this case the correlation coefficient is represented by τ_b and is given by the formula:

$$\tau_b = \frac{S}{\frac{1}{2}\sqrt{(N^2 - \Sigma t_i^2)(N^2 - \Sigma u_i^2)}}$$

where t_i represents the total number of individuals at each rank for variable A, and u_i the corresponding value for variable B. (The above formula reduces to that for τ_a when there are no ties,

174

since then all values of t_i and u_i are unity, and $\Sigma t_i^2 = \Sigma u_i^2 = N$.)

Where the extent or the distribution of ties is different in the two rank orders, however, τ_b has two disadvantages: (i) it may not be able to attain unity, and therefore (ii) two different but fairly close values of τ_b may not be comparable, the larger not necessarily representing the higher correlation. In these cases only the value of p, the probability of attaining or exceeding this value of τ_b by chance alone, can be used for comparison. These two disadvantages have to be accepted.

τ has the following advantages for the present study:

1. It does not depend on the assumption that there is an underlying continuously varying quantity on which the two rank orders are based. (This advantage is not shared by the Product-Moment Correlation Coefficient.)
2. It is applicable to any $r \times s$ contingency table, where r and s need not be equal and may have any value from two upwards.
3. Provided that N is greater than 10, the probability (p) of attaining or exceeding any given value of τ_a or τ_b by chance alone can be calculated with reasonable accuracy. (This advantage is not shared by Spearman's Rank Correlation Coefficient when there is a high proportion of ties in either of the two rank orders.)

DIFFERENT FORMS OF HYPOTHESIS

This leads at once to the very important question of *different forms of hypothesis*, an exposition of which is essential to clear thinking about the present work. The problem which will be repeatedly under consideration is the study of some factor X in these therapies in relation to outcome. Now a correlation coefficient such as τ gives a test of what I call the *hypothesis of parallel variation*, which takes the form:

The more a factor X is present, the more favourable does the outcome tend to be.

The implication is, partly, that X is both a *necessary* and a *sufficient* condition to success.

A limiting case of this kind of hypothesis is thus the *hypothesis of the necessary and sufficient condition*:

If X is present outcome tends to be favourable; if X is absent, unfavourable.

175

The present work

The confirmation of this hypothesis requires that:

(a) of successful therapies a high proportion contains X, and
(b) of unsuccessful therapies a high proportion does not contain X.

This is best illustrated by means of the 2×2 contingency table:

	X	
Outcome	*Present*	*Absent*
Favourable		
Unfavourable		

An exact figure for the probability of a given distribution (the Fisher test) can be obtained from tables.

Now in fact, clinically speaking, it seems highly unlikely that any factor would be found which would be both a necessary and a sufficient condition to success. There is, then, a third type of hypothesis which may be of far more clinical value, the *hypothesis of the necessary condition*, simply:

X is a necessary condition to success.

This requires for its confirmation that:

(a) of the *successful therapies* a high proportion contains X; and
(b) of the *therapies that do not contain X* a high proportion is unsuccessful; while
(c) therapies that *contain X* and are yet *unsuccessful* (those in the bottom left-hand corner of the diagram above) are *irrelevant*.

The difference in form between requirements (a) and (b) gives the result that this type of hypothesis cannot be tested by any correlation coefficient, unless the proportion of cases in the bottom left-hand corner happens to be small. In fact, however, the correlation coefficient therefore gives a *highly conservative* test for this type of hypothesis—unless the cases in the top right-hand corner greatly outnumber those in the bottom left-hand corner—and will for this reason be used here. It must always be remembered that 'exceptions' of the 'X present—failure' category have far less weight than those of the 'X absent—success' category; but at the same time that there must be a reasonable

176

proportion of both the categories 'X present—success' and 'X absent—failure' to make the test meaningful.

After this long preliminary, we are in a position to use these methods in order to test the first of the classes of actual factor represented by X, namely selection criteria.

CHAPTER 9

Selection Criteria

During the preliminary discussion and later work many ideas about selection criteria were put forward, mainly by Balint, but here consideration will be confined to those on which the evidence is fairly clear.

The two main hypotheses were exactly similar to those found in the literature, namely the relatively 'static' Hypothesis A:

> That the prognosis is best in *mild illnesses* of relatively *recent onset*;

and the more 'dynamic' Hypothesis B:

> That the prognosis is best in those patients who show evidence from the beginning of a willingness and an ability to *work in interpretative therapy.*

As discussed on pp. 21 and 26–7, both these hypotheses can be broken down into more than one factor. Hypothesis A contains:

Criterion 1: 'Mild and circumscribed psychopathology' (in psycho-analytic terms, particularly 'genital level', 'three-person', or 'Oedipal' problems; rather than 'oral level', 'two-person', 'primitive', or 'deeply depressive' problems).

Criterion 2: 'Sound basic personality.'

Criterion 3: 'History of satisfactory personal relationships.'

Criterion 4: 'Recent onset.'

An alternative to Criterion 4 is Criterion 5, 'Propitious moment': a moment in a relatively chronic illness felt to be especially favourable because of external or internal factors. An example is provided by the Storm Lady who—though she had suffered from her symptom for as long as she could remember—was now pregnant for the first time and felt it was essential to get help before she had her baby.

Hypothesis B also contains more than one factor:

Criterion 6: 'High motivation for therapy.'
Criterion 7: 'Good contact with the interviewer and at least some response to interpretation.'

SELECTION OF PATIENTS

The requirement for a valid experiment is that the series of patients treated should include a sufficient number of patients thought to be *unsuitable*, to act as 'controls'. If we had been able to hold to our original aim of selecting only 'suitable' patients, we would now be in no position to say very much about selection criteria at all. In fact this aim was nullified by an ecological process impelled by powerful forces. The two most important of these were, first, that apparently suitable patients were very much rarer than we had supposed. The vast majority of patients referred to the Tavistock Clinic are suffering from chronic character problems. The second factor was that when this group of enthusiastic therapists was put together with this population of patients, the processes of interaction became almost autonomous and were far too strong for many of the restraints imposed by the purpose of the work. The patient's desperate need for treatment (Tom), the interest of the case (Storm Lady), the intense relation formed—on both sides—between patient and therapist at interview (Paranoid Engineer), the need of a therapist to prove himself to the group on his first case (Neurasthenic's Husband), all played their part in selection. The final result was a population of patients containing—quite by chance—almost equal numbers of patients with a good, an intermediate, and a poor prognosis— in fact, exactly what a group of disciplined scientists should have provided. (Unfortunately the opinions expressed by different members of the Workshop on the same patient are so heterogeneous that I have not found it possible to study the relation between implied prognosis and outcome in any convincing way.)

Yet it is quite essential to emphasize that this series of patients still forms a *very highly selected population*, and some statement should be made of the characteristics of this population, as far as they can be recognized.

The patients accepted for consultation at the Tavistock Clinic can really be described as the 'cream' of the whole London area as far as 'suitability' for psychotherapy can be judged at all. This

179

does not mean that they do not contain members of the 'working class' or patients of only average intelligence, but it does mean that they are weighted in favour of the 'professional classes' and people with a high capacity for insight. Our own population, selected from these, consisted almost entirely of patients of whom it could be said:

1. they were willing and able to explore their feelings;
2. they were judged to be capable of working within a therapeutic relationship based on interpretation;
3. by the end of the assessment period, they made us feel that we understood the nature of their 'real' problems in dynamic terms;
4. with each, therefore, we were able to formulate some kind of circumscribed therapeutic plan which—as far as we could judge—seemed feasible at the time.

When the rough scores for individual criteria are inspected, certain other characteristics emerge:

5. fourteen of the nineteen patients in the present study (i.e. omitting those for whom the outcome cannot be scored) were judged to have been taken on at a 'propitious moment' (Criterion 5);
6. twelve of the nineteen were judged to have a 'sound basic personality' (Criterion 2).

Finally, though severely 'ill' patients were included (e.g. the Paranoid Engineer and the Hypertensive Housewife), it is possible to imagine patients much more severely ill or much more obviously unsuitable who were not included and who certainly would not have been considered—psychopaths, frank psychotics, malignant hysterics, severely self-destructive characters, or patients likely to make a determined attempt at suicide. No patient, for instance, had ever—when first accepted—been admitted to hospital because of mental illness; and, when accepted, every patient was either at work or running a home (the Student's Wife had been forced by her symptoms to leave work, but was still running a home; Tom had just left school). Thus, for the following criteria: nature of psychopathology (1), response to interpretation (7), and even motivation (6), it is variations in the 'upper' end of the scale—in other words 'fine' rather than 'gross' effects—that are being studied. All these considerations are very important, because they mean that our study is almost certainly not comparable with many of those listed in *Table 3*; and therefore, where apparently different conclusions are reached, our conclusions and those of other authors do not necessarily conflict.

Of the five criteria contained in this hypothesis, only two are suitable for study in our data: nature of psychopathology (1), and recent onset (4).

Criterion 1: Nature of Psychopathology

The approach used for the study of this criterion will be entirely clinical.

First of all, there were included in this series two patients who were known at assessment to be very ill, the Paranoid Engineer (latent paranoid psychosis) and the Hypertensive Housewife (severe depression). To these should certainly be added Tom, whose subsequent history revealed a much more severe illness than was originally realized—either an exceptionally crippling anxiety-hysteria or else a borderline psychosis; and possibly the Storm Lady, who—although a much better preserved personality —suffered beneath her lifelong monosymptomatic phobia from the kind of phantasies that appear in severe depression. In all four of these, brief psychotherapy was a clear-cut failure.

Yet the next stage of 'severity'—the complex or extensive character problems, and the symptomatic illnesses masking such problems—will be found at once to contain most of our best results (four out of five of those that score 3). The most striking is of course the Neurasthenic's Husband. The following are quotations from the psychiatrist's and the psychologist's reports on this case:

Psychiatrist (*the therapist*): 'This man's masochism . . . his impotence and homosexuality, his need to be degraded, suggest a massive personality disturbance. This is, however, in contrast with his work record, which is progressive, as long as it is done under the shelter of a strong organization.'

Psychologist: 'Mr. X appears to be a bizarre character, possibly fairly well stabilized. The anxieties against which he is defending himself appear to have a psychotic element and he may become much less stable under treatment.

He is depressed, schizoid, uses mechanisms of detachment and obsessional verbalization. . . .'[1]

[1] The report of the psychologist, who was not a member of the Workshop, is almost certainly exaggerated; but it gives some indication of just how unsuitable for psychotherapy this patient appeared to be.

181

The present work

Similarly, on the Biologist:

Report by interviewing psychiatrist (not a Workshop member): 'He puts on a very presentable front, behind which in fact very much more neurosis exists than might be suspected. He is in fact very much more disturbed than appears, but his controlling mechanisms are very well developed.'

Extract from Discussion:
> *Balint*: 'Hysterical presenting symptom in a mainly obsessional character.'
> *Psychologist*: 'With a paranoid element.'

And on the Falling Social Worker:

Extract from Discussion:
> *Balint*: 'By the material, I would say that it might be a very nice five-year analysis. It's not that the woman is not suitable for therapy, but whether she is suitable for our kind of therapy?'

Finally, although the Lighterman was felt at discussion to be a highly suitable case, he was revealed by therapy to have been suffering from severe compulsiveness affecting his whole life for many years, and beneath this lay an essentially depressive illness.

The other patients originally judged to be suffering from relatively severe problems or character problems are: the Unsuccessful Accountant (score 1 for outcome); Violet's Mother and the Student's Wife (score 0).

At the other end of the scale, those patients who at assessment appeared to be not very 'ill' and to be suffering from relatively 'simple' 'Oedipal' problems provided only one score of 3 for outcome (the Railway Solicitor), one score of 2 (the Girl with the Dreams), one of 1 (the Civil Servant), and two of 0 (the Draper's Assistant and the Articled Accountant). The Surgeon's Daughter (score 1) should be added to this list because, although at assessment she appeared to be suffering from a complex illness, in fact she was probably one of the least ill of all, and her psychopathology was relatively simple. The Student Thief (score 0) is omitted, since the severity of her psychopathology is still uncertain; and the Pilot's Wife (score 0) also, because of the uncertain mutual influence of her psychopathological and endocrine conditions.

Although the numbers are very small, it will be seen that the best therapeutic results tended to come not from the apparently mild and simple illnesses, but from those judged to be of intermediate severity and complexity. In other words, the aspect of

182

Hypothesis A concerned with psychopathology is not confirmed; that is, unless the line of demarcation between 'suitable' and 'unsuitable' patients is placed much nearer to the 'severe' end of the scale than all previous statements of this hypothesis, including our own, would predict.

It should be added that there is one factor not included in the original hypotheses which may possibly indicate a bad prognosis. This is *serious quarrelling between the parents*, which may be seen from the entries under Home Atmosphere in the Assessment and Therapy Forms. It occurred in the case of one patient who scored 1 for outcome (the Surgeon's Daughter); three who scored 0 (the Storm Lady, the Student Thief, Tom); and the two with no score in whom therapy cannot be regarded as having had more than a very limited success (the Clown, the Dog Lady). The figures are of course too small to be more than suggestive.

Criterion 4: Recent Onset
This criterion can be treated by a purely statistical method because definite figures are available in the clinical notes. The evidence is shown in *Table 9*.

TABLE 9 CRITERION 4: ONSET OF SYMPTOMS—OUTCOME
General criteria of scoring

(a) It is the patient's complaint that is considered. The 'real' problem is ignored.

(b) Onset less than 1 year ago: score 2
      1-4 years ago: score 1
      more than 4 years ago: score 0

Patient	Score for outcome	Score for onset	Rationale for scoring
Biologist	3	1	Eating phobia, acute onset, $3\frac{1}{2}$ years.
Lighterman	3	2	Anxiety, acute onset, 2–3 months.
Neurasthenic's Husband	3	0	On the waiting list for psycho-analysis 15 years.
Falling Social Worker	3	0 (or 1 ?)	Phobias, mild 10 years, increasing 4 years; recent acute exacerbation.
Railway Solicitor	3	1	Headaches, fairly acute onset, $2\frac{1}{2}$ years.

Table 9—*continued*

Patient	Score for outcome	Score for onset	Rationale for Scoring
Girl with the Dreams	2	2 or 1	Disturbing dreams, lack of concentration, 'a number of years'; acute panic attack, 2 months.
Civil Servant	1	2	Agoraphobia, eating phobia; acute onset, 6 months.
Surgeon's Daughter	1	2?	Unmarried pregnancy; though she also asked help for 'background problems', presumably of long duration.
Unsuccessful Accountant	1	1	Inability to get a job for 2 years.
Draper's Assistant	0	2	Non-consummation after 7 months of marriage.
Storm Lady	0	0	Lifelong fear of death; storm phobia mainly for 3 years.
Tom	0	2	Anxiety attacks, acute onset, 4 weeks.
Hypertensive Housewife	0	1	Depression, 4 years.
Pilot's Wife	0	2	Frigidity after 10 months of marriage.
Student Thief	0	1 or 2	Stealing 1–2 weeks ago admitted; possibly stealing for 1 or 2 years
Paranoid Engineer	0	0	Homosexual feelings for at least 5 years; gradual onset; recent severe exacerbation.
Violet's Mother	0	–	Patient made no complaints about herself.
Articled Accountant	0	2	Acute homosexual breakdown, 8 weeks.
Student's Wife	0	2	Phobias, acute onset, 11 months.

The scoring is deliberately chosen to provide the highest possible correlation (e.g. the line of demarcation between a score of 1 and a score of 0 is set at four years in order to give a score of 1 rather than 0 to two successful cases, the Biologist and the Railway Solicitor). Even so, and even if the 'best' possible scores are chosen where there is some doubt (the Falling Social Worker, 1; the Girl with the Dreams, 2; the Student Thief, 1), the value of τ_b is slightly negative. I can only add that a clinical scrutiny of the figures fails to reveal any reason why this purely statistical result should not be accepted.

Finally, a clinical study of a combination of Criteria (1) and (4) fails equally to reveal any correlation with successful outcome.

Summary of Evidence on Hypothesis A
The evidence from this small population of patients suggests:

1. That if 'mildness' of psychopathology and recent onset of symptoms do exert any favourable influence on outcome, then this influence is much less important than that of other factors.

2. That the point at which 'severity' and 'extensiveness' of psychopathology begin to exert an appreciable unfavourable influence lies far nearer to the severe and extensive end of the scale than Hypothesis A, as usually stated, would suggest.

Obviously, the failure of the hypothesis is therapy's gain.

EVIDENCE ON HYPOTHESIS B

In view of this result, it is natural to turn to the two criteria of Hypothesis B, motivation and response to interpretation, both of which are completely independent of the psychopathology. Of the two, little case can be made out in favour of the second. This is largely because the ability to work in interpretative therapy, which usually implies some sort of response to interpretation, was regarded as a necessary condition to accepting a patient for treatment. The result is a relative absence of 'controls', which —however important this criterion may be—makes its testing quite impossible.

It has always seemed to me, in the course of several years of study, that the one remaining criterion, motivation, offered the only hope of being of value. The way of presenting the evidence for this, and the exact form of the hypothesis put forward, have passed through several different stages. Because of the discovery of some contrary evidence, the original hypothesis has had to be modified.

The present work

It is first necessary to consider exactly what is meant by motivation. The obvious aspect of motivation which is likely to come to mind is simply the strength of the wish to come for treatment; but further thought will show that this can be only a part of what is important—clearly the patient must also want the kind of treatment that he is being offered. Now, in our kind of approach, it will be made fairly plain to him at consultation that what he will be offered is insight, and that if he is asking for something else he will not receive it. His true motivation will then be shown in whether he still wants to come and whether it is really insight that he is seeking. This latter aspect of motivation was embodied in one of Balint's criteria, that 'the therapist's and patient's aims must be the same'.

There is, however, a serious difficulty here. A phenomenon universally experienced in dynamic therapy is resistance. This means that every patient's motivation for insight, and many patients' motivation to come, are ambivalent, containing both a positive and a negative component. Moreover, marked fluctuations in motivation occur regularly in therapy, especially during the initial stages. In fact, in all but three of the patients in the present series, evidence for both components of motivation can be found. Now presumably the aspect of motivation requiring study is the balance between the two. But this is extremely difficult to judge even prospectively, and it is almost impossible to keep retrospective judgements free of contamination by knowledge of the outcome. Consequently no formal scoring is possible; though quite convincing (if rather complicated) evidence, based entirely on the written records, can nevertheless be presented.

Since it has become clear that the same tendencies are present in the next series of patients treated, and since unequivocal evidence for motivation can be obtained in only a certain proportion of either series, I have combined the two, adding nine patients from the second series (out of fifteen) in whom reasonably certain judgements of outcome can be made. The main fluctuations in motivation seem to occur during the first four or five sessions; and for the present purposes this is taken as the 'initial period' of therapy, during which the evidence for motivation in these patients will be studied.

Now it is probably true that, although there were a number of patients with high motivation who scored 0 for outcome, the data (statistically) support the hypothesis of parallel variation—the higher the motivation the better the outcome. Nevertheless, since reliable scoring is quite impossible, a less exacting hypothesis will

186

be put forward, and this will be supported by evidence only from two extreme ends of the scale—namely from those patients who scored 3 for outcome and from those who had in my judgement the lowest motivation. These are the patients most relevant to the hypothesis that 'high motivation is a necessary condition to a score of 3 for outcome'.

For clarity, the evidence will be summarized before being presented in detail.

Of the seven patients (five in the present series; two in the second) who scored 3 for outcome:

(a) One (the Falling Social Worker) showed a high positive component of motivation without any evidence for a negative component.

(b) Two (the Lighterman and Mr. M) showed a high initial motivation with a temporary decrease in session 4.

(c) Two (the Biologist and Mrs. C_1) showed a low initial motivation with an immediate increase after their first experience of an interpretative situation.

(d) One (the Neurasthenic's Husband) showed an exceptionally high motivation before interview; but at interview and for several sessions afterwards showed a distaste for painful interpretations, and failed to attend on one occasion (session 4).

(e) One (the Railway Solicitor) was judged by the therapist to have a high initial motivation; but, though he showed no actual distaste for insight, he provided evidence later that he might really be seeking something else.

(f) A complication in the evidence is that four of the above patients (the Lighterman, Mr. M, the Neurasthenic's Husband, and the Railway Solicitor) showed a clear temporary decrease in motivation in session 4 or 5.

Although the evidence for high motivation in the above patients is thus by no means unequivocal, at least seven other patients can be found (four in the present series; three in the second) in whom the balance of motivation seems to have been considerably lower even than in the Neurasthenic's Husband and the Railway Solicitor; and of these seven, six scored 0 for outcome. This balance of motivation can be brought out very clearly by a comparison of the patients' actual behaviour. Thus it is clear that a patient who is at least willing to give treatment a trial and is asking for help for himself (as was true of all the above patients)

187

must probably be judged to have a higher motivation than one who spends four or five sessions wondering whether to come or not (Mr. Y_1, Mr. J_2), or than one who comes asking for advice about her family and shows a persistent distaste for examining her own problems at all (Violet's Mother); and also that one who simply misses one weekly session (the Neurasthenic's Husband) must be judged to have a higher motivation than one who stays away for six months (the Pilot's Wife), or for six weeks and then has to be *sent* back (the Student Thief), or than one who breaks off treatment altogether (Tom, Mr. Y_2).

The detailed evidence will now be presented:

Patients who scored 3 for outcome

(*a*) *The Biologist.* This patient showed unequivocal evidence for fairly high motivation to come in that, having asked for an appointment to be given to him after his return from holiday, he waited for three weeks without hearing, and then wrote: 'I am surprised not to have had another letter from you. . . . I should be most grateful if you could arrange another consultation at your earliest convenience.' Some doubt can be cast on this, however, because there were external reasons for his seeking an appointment soon, since he probably knew by that time that he had only a few more months in London.

His original motivation for insight was low. In his Rorschach interview he told the psychologist that he remained to be convinced that his problem was psychological. The psychologist did some interpretative work, and the opening words of the report on session 1 are: 'He has come to the view that his problems are psychological.' He then almost at once plunged into what seemed to be the heart of his problem, namely his relations with men.

Summary: Objective evidence for fairly high motivation to come and for a marked increase in motivation for insight after his first contact with interpretations.

(*b*) *The Lighterman.* Here the written evidence is rather indirect and not entirely satisfactory, but it fits in with the therapist's retrospective judgement of high motivation. The patient's fairly high motivation to come is indicated by the fact that since he was in a crisis the therapist offered him the first four appointments within seven days, and he came willingly to all of these. His high motivation for insight is suggested by the fact that although he had had no previous contact with psychological thinking he was

188

already working out interpretations for himself in session 2. There was a moment of flagging motivation in session 4, when he seemed to be saying that he would be glad to be released from the treatment, and in fact he decided to try to manage on his own for a fortnight. But in session 5 he clearly seemed 'to be asking for a further interpretation' and intense therapy began again.

Summary: Indirect evidence for high motivation both to come and for insight, though with a moment of flagging motivation in session 4.

(*c*) *The Neurasthenic's Husband.* The way in which this patient obtained treatment gives unequivocal evidence of, initially, an extremely high positive component of motivation both to come and for insight. He had been on the waiting list of psycho-analysis for fifteen years without being offered a vacancy. He finally wrote a letter to the clinic, from which the following is an extract: 'An urge has come over me to throw away what is useless [in the house] . . . to let the air and light in . . . this urge must be complementary to my wish to clean up the dark corners of my own soul . . . I am stressing, perhaps overstressing, the hopefulness of this moment, but I cannot overstate the case for the urgency.'

As soon as he was subjected to interpretation, however, the negative component of his motivation was revealed as also very strong. The therapist wrote '. . . but if I interrupted and touched on some difficult topic he either nodded his head in masochistic agreement, or said I was quite wrong and went on with his story.' He was described by the therapist as 'not very sincere' after session 3; and finally he failed to attend for session 4, which the therapist attributed to the fact that in session 3 the difficult subject of anger had been touched on. He came back the next week and therapy was resumed.

Summary: Objective evidence that the motivation to come and for insight were at first extremely high, but dropped rapidly to a low level in face of painful interpretations.

(*d*) *The Falling Social Worker.* Here there are two clinical judgements of high motivation. (i) The psychiatric social worker wrote: '[She] left me in no doubt that she had sought psychiatric help of her own accord, feeling it to be the only treatment which could help her.' (ii) After session 1 the therapist wrote: 'She seemed to me to have a fair capacity for response to interpretation and a strong drive towards recovery.'

189

The present work

After interpretations in session 1, this patient succeeded in telling the therapist some things of which she was ashamed, and which she had not dared to tell her previous therapist during therapeutic contact lasting a total of three years.

This is one of the very few patients in whom no evidence for a negative component of motivation can be found.

Summary: Evidence, based on judgements made at the time, for high motivation for therapy; with some objective evidence of ability to face painful feelings. No evidence for a negative component to motivation.

(*e*) *The Railway Solicitor*. Of these seven patients who scored 3 for outcome, the evidence for motivation is most doubtful in this patient. The therapist wrote after session 1: ' . . . he shows a considerable capacity for insight . . . and a strong desire to get well, which, however, might lead him into a flight into health very quickly.' At discussion the Workshop was divided about his motivation. Balint said (with reference to his motivation for insight) that 'everything the interviewer said was taken seriously'; while Main (with reference to his motivation to come) questioned whether he had been pushed into therapy by the referring psychiatrist.

Later evidence suggested that it might be something other than insight that he was seeking. The following is from the therapist's remarks at discussion after session 4: 'The most important part of all the sessions occurs in the last two minutes. During the course of the session he asks me questions and I try to deal with what it means, and he rather glibly picks up what I am saying. At the end he says, "By the way, doctor, about the questions I asked you, would you give me an answer" . . . I don't really feel my interpretations go home in terms of his doing any work. . . . The whole forty-five minutes of the session he is playing with me until the last minutes when he wants to get something.' The therapist's prediction of an attempted flight into health was in fact confirmed in session 5, in which the patient said he was very pleased with his progress and felt he could leave treatment in a week or two. The hypomanic element in this became clear in session 6.

Summary: Explicit judgement made by therapist after session 1 of high motivation both to come and for insight; but this contradicted by objective evidence that he was seeking something other than insight.

(*f*) *Mrs. C₁* (*score for outcome probably 3*). This patient's initial motivation was low, as is shown by the fact that she had been advised to seek psychotherapy for her frigidity but had delayed for a year before doing so.

When she was finally seen for consultation the interviewer wrote that a particular interpretation 'made a considerable impression on her . . . and from then on we went immediately over to possible therapeutic help'. Thereafter, all the evidence indicated that her motivation was strong. The psychologist who saw her next wrote: 'She earnestly wants help and is able to make use of a [therapeutic] relationship.' There was then a delay of one month before interview and test came to discussion, from which the following is an extract: 'Mrs. Balint is impressed by the fact that the woman is keen for treatment and has rung up since [her initial interview] asking when it will begin.'

There is no contrary evidence.

Summary: Objective evidence for initially low motivation, changing to uniformly high motivation after a single interpretative interview.

(*g*) *Mr. M* (*score for outcome definitely 3*). This patient's high motivation to come was shown by his saying at interview that 'when he got the original letter from us saying that there might be a long delay before he could be seen he had got very depressed, and when he had got the letter mentioning the present appointment his depression had got much better'.

He was next seen for a projection test. The same day he wrote a long letter to the original interviewer, consisting largely of free associations, and describing a number of things that he had felt in the test but had not been able to bring himself to say. In other words, he tried to start therapy before he had yet been taken on.

He did, however, show a marked flagging of motivation in a later session (no. 4) in which he said that: '. . . he had very much been wondering about the future and whether he wanted to stay where he was or go wandering.' He made a clear response to the interpretation that he wanted to break off relationships, including that with the therapist, as soon as something started to go wrong. This in fact was his central problem appearing in the transference.

Summary: Objective evidence for high initial motivation, increasing further after a single interpretative interview, but with a fall in motivation in session 4.

The present work

Patients who showed the lowest motivation

(a) *Mr. Y_1 (score 1-2 for outcome)*. This patient revealed a remarkable ambivalence in his motivation. He repeatedly showed reluctance to accept treatment, but the moment he was faced with the prospect of not coming he would start to communicate about the centre of his problem. This happened in sessions 1, 2, and 5, and the therapist was consequently unable to lay down a programme for therapy till session 5. In this session, in fact, the therapist at first more or less agreed to let the patient terminate, but 'the moment this was agreed he started to communicate and the session ended up by being unquestionably the most important so far'.

Summary: Prolonged hesitation about accepting treatment, though with evidence for a strong positive as well as a strong negative component of motivation. According to my judgement this patient showed on balance a higher motivation than any of the six that follow.

(b) *Tom (score 0 for outcome)*. This boy's initial motivation to come was extremely high, as is shown by the following from session 2: 'I [therapist] remark on his glancing at the clock as a wish that the session would end so that we would not have to examine these upsetting things any further.' [Patient] 'Not at all; I have put everything into treatment here. . . . Got to get to work in a week or so; there is not much time to get better. Need help very much.'

Yet it was also clear from the beginning that his motivation for insight was ambivalent. The interviewer wrote: 'Tom's emotional attitude to his symptoms varies between feeling that they might be bound up with emotional problems and falling back on the defence that they are purely physical.' The negative component in his motivation had completely got the upper hand by session 4, in which Tom reported that he had solved his problem by going to live with his stepmother: 'I [therapist] . . . try to get him to look more closely at his feelings about father. He remains obstinate, saying that he has gone to live with mother to get himself well, and he will never get well if he keeps on thinking about all these problems. Nothing I could do could produce any change.' He then broke off treatment and refused to return.

Summary: Evidence for very high motivation to come but ambivalent motivation for insight; motivation decreasing to zero after 4 sessions, so that patient breaks off treatment.

(*c*) *The Pilot's Wife* (*score 0 for outcome*). This patient's behaviour at first showed that her overall motivation to come, though ambivalent, was fairly high. A condensed quotation from the report on the initial interview is as follows: 'The ambivalence came out fairly strongly in favour of treatment. She said she did not believe in psychiatry, but if I felt I could help her she would come. It appeared that she was willing to take some trouble to come—she was going to a new job, but she felt she would be able to give up her lunch hour or come here at 9 o'clock in the morning so that she did not lose very much time. When asked if she wanted to make a definite appointment she said yes. This wish for treatment is in her favour.'

The remark about 'not believing in psychiatry' suggests that her motivation for insight was not very high, and this was confirmed when in session 2 she proceeded to do nothing but make polite conversation, and got resentful when this was pointed out.

Then: 'Five minutes before session 3 she rang up and said that her husband had got into trouble and she would have to jump on the nearest train. I [therapist] asked if she wanted another appointment but she said could we leave it.'

Nothing further was heard for six months, when the referring doctor wrote to the therapist asking if she could be given another appointment. The patient wrote that her husband's trouble had been cleared up seven weeks ago 'but, after such a long pause, I felt too embarrassed to approach you. So I waited until my annual check-up at the local family planning clinic in order to explain my predicament [to the referring doctor]. . . . I am anxious to undergo treatment if possible.'

In fact, from then on, there was no doubt of her strong motivation to come; and, against great resistance, of her motivation for insight.

Summary: Ambivalent, giving at first objective evidence of high motivation to come; and then objective evidence of very low motivation; finally high motivation once more.

(*d*) *The Student Thief* (*score 0 for outcome*). This patient was sent for treatment by her matron after she had admitted to two thefts, and this method of referral must at once cast doubt on her motivation. She arrived fifteen minutes late for her first appointment at the clinic. The psychologist, who saw her next, said: 'She can hardly wait to see the therapist again, she was helped so much.' However, when she was seen in fact, she 'implied she didn't really want to come' for treatment, though she also 'jumped at' an appointment offered for three weeks ahead. In fact she failed to attend for this appointment, and when asked about this later she said that she had not felt 'composed enough' to come, after her fiancé's departure abroad. She was not heard from again for another three weeks, after which she was once more sent for treatment by her matron because of the discovery of two further thefts. Her motivation continued ambivalent—although she seemed deeply involved in therapy and said she could not manage without it, she repeatedly arrived late for sessions (once by as much as forty minutes) without apology.

Summary: Much objective evidence for low motivation, including considerable acting out over appointments.

(*e*) *Violet's Mother* (*score 0 for outcome*). There is abundant evidence in the clinical notes that this patient wanted a number of things from the therapist which did not include insight into her own problems. In session 1: 'For the first threequarters of an hour she insisted on talking about [her family's] problems entirely.' The therapist eventually made contact with her own unhappiness and she asked if she could come back. Nevertheless in session 2 it seemed that what she wanted was 'guidance and support' (therapist's words); in session 3 'instruction' (patient's word); in session 4: 'The essential point of this session was the divergence of what she and I wanted from the treatment. It was quite clear that she wanted definite instruction about how she could handle the situation at home.'

Even her motivation to come was low, e.g. between sessions 2 and 3 she said (on 11 December) 'that she had not felt very well after the last interview . . . so could she put off seeing me until after Christmas'.

Summary: Abundant objective evidence of very low motivation for insight and low motivation to come.

(*f*) *Mr. J₂* (*score 0 for outcome, follow-up 15 months*). This patient had a 'black-out' after an emotional crisis with his fiancée, and was advised to seek treatment by his fiancée and by the casualty officer who saw him. As might be expected from this way of coming for treatment, his own motivation was at first very low, and he hesitated for several sessions before finally accepting treatment. One of his defences was to try to concentrate on his fiancée's difficulties rather than on his own. This appeared in session 2,

194

in which 'he did not seem to be asking for more help', but 'asked if it would be possible for his fiancée to see someone'; in session 3, 'whenever I tried to talk about him his associations quickly veered away to talking about his fiancée and her contribution to the present troubles'; and in session 4, 'I pointed out to him that he seemed quite willing to look at his fiancée's difficulties rather than his own'. It was only in sessions 4 and 5 that any real contact could be made with his feelings, and a programme for therapy could not be laid down till the end of session 5.

Summary: Extensive objective evidence for low motivation both to come and for insight.

(g) *Mr. Y_2 (assumed score 0, no follow-up)*. This patient had a consultation with a non-Workshop psychiatrist and a test with a Workshop psychologist, and was then seen by the therapist, who reported as follows: 'There seems to be no urgency about his problem but instead he is seeking for information about what sort of treatment he will get. Talk treatment (?). Hypnosis (?). He seems to be seeking the latter.' The report on session 2 states: 'He wanted me to cure him by magic and did not accept the discussion or take part in it.'

After session 3 he wrote asking if further sessions could be postponed, and saying that nothing seemed to have been achieved. 'I confess I am sometimes a little bored. This is why I think a rest would be useful.' He promised to get in touch with the therapist in the future but has not done so. There was no evidence for any improvement.

Summary: Very low motivation for insight from the beginning; motivation to come fell to zero after session 3.

Various aspects of the evidence provided by these fourteen patients (out of a total of twenty-eight) may now be summarized and discussed:

1. At least six out of seven (86 per cent) of the patients who scored 3 for outcome (the possible exception being the Railway Solicitor) showed either (a) a very high initial positive component of motivation both to come and for insight, or (b) a marked increase in motivation in response to their first experience of interpretative therapy.

2. The six patients (out of fifteen, 40 per cent) who, according to my judgement, showed on balance the lowest motivation in the

195

two series combined, *all* scored 0 for outcome. None of these six patients showed a high positive component of motivation for insight.

3. The aspect of motivation that may turn out to be the most reliable indicator of a poor prognosis is *acting out over appointments*—obviously, if it results in breaking off treatment (Tom, Mr. Y$_2$); or if it is shown in the missing of a session (the Pilot's Wife, the Student Thief), or in the postponement of a session (Violet's Mother). The only patient who scored 3 and behaved thus was the Neurasthenic's Husband (who missed session 4), and in him the positive component of motivation was exceptionally high. Two other patients (the Dog Lady and Miss T), who have been omitted because of uncertainty in the therapeutic result, showed the most persistent acting out of all. In both of these it is doubtful if the improvement observed qualifies for a score as high as 1. It should be added that the Student Thief (score 0) arrived late (by a quarter of an hour) for her initial appointment at the clinic; and two other patients who scored 0 but were not included in the above evidence did the same, namely the Draper's Assistant (quarter of an hour) and Mr. W (twenty-five minutes). There is no record that any of the other patients did so. The Draper's Assistant also lost the letter offering her the appointment for her first therapeutic session, and only rang up at the last moment to say that she would come. One patient who scored 2 (Mr. C$_2$) came ten minutes late to sessions 3 and 4. (Cancellation of sessions for reasons presumably beyond the patient's control is not included here.)

4. The remarkable prevalence of a decrease in motivation in sessions 3 to 5, not only in patients who scored 0 for outcome but also in those who scored 3, is of great interest. This is summarized in *Table 10* on page 197.

To this list should be added the Articled Accountant (score 0) whose initial motivation seemed to be extremely high, but who admitted in session 3 that 'He did not want to go on, and really wanted to forget the whole thing'; and Mr. C$_2$ (score 2) who, as already mentioned, came late for sessions 3 and 4.

This phenomenon was noted by Vosburg (1958) in a study of the case notes of therapies conducted by psychiatric residents:

'In the first three hours [i.e. interviews], an initial history of the patient is taken, and the patient invariably reacts to his disclosures with strong feelings. Apparently because of these feelings, two-thirds of the patients either cancel or are late

196

TABLE 10 EVIDENCE FOR EARLY DECREASE IN MOTIVATION

Patient	Outcome	Evidence for decrease in motivation	Session no.
Lighterman	3	Tries to manage on his own.	4
Neurasthenic's Husband	3	Fails to attend.	4
Railway Solicitor	3	Attempts flight into health.	5
Mr. M	3	Would 'like to go wandering again'.	4
Tom	0	Breaks off treatment.	4
Pilot's Wife	0	Postpones treatment for six months.	3
Student Thief	0	Fails to attend; stays away three further weeks.	3
Violet's Mother	0	Postpones session for three weeks.	3
Mr. Y_2	0	Breaks off treatment.	3

about the third interview. It would seem that this development is an *initial crisis* of psychotherapy.'

It is possible that the characteristics of this falling off in motivation may have prognostic value, since in our cases that scored 0 for outcome it tended on the whole to occur from an initially lower motivation, more markedly, and earlier than in those that scored 3.

5. It is worth adding some marginal evidence from one patient, the Paranoid Engineer. He probably had the highest motivation of all these patients—he was living on a very low salary and said that he had saved just £50 and wanted to spend it on 25 sessions. There was no evidence whatsoever for a negative component in his motivation. Although the immediate outcome in this case was failure to terminate, the final outcome of some seventy sessions

during three years certainly merits a score of 3—and this in spite of the fact that this patient, being a borderline psychotic, was almost certainly the most severely ill in the two series combined.

The foregoing evidence will thus be seen to support (statistically rather than absolutely) the following hypotheses, which apply to the 'initial period' of therapy—here taken to be the first four or five sessions:

1. That a high initial positive component of motivation both to come and for insight, or a marked increase in motivation following exposure to an interpretative situation, is a necessary condition to a score of 3 for outcome.

2. That a very low motivation, or a further decrease from an initially low motivation, especially if indicated by acting out over appointments, predicts a score of 0 for outcome.

3. On the other hand, that an early decrease from an initially high motivation—even if marked—is quite compatible with a score of 3 for outcome.

The clinical meaning of 2 and 3 is presumably that, whereas resistance is almost inevitable, only a high underlying motivation will carry a patient successfully through it.

It will also be clear that in these hypotheses the two criteria of Hypothesis B are combined—in that emphasis is laid not only on motivation itself, but also on the changes in motivation that occur in response to interpretation.

Since further suggestions about selection criteria are put forward on pp. 213 and 276–7 below, further discussion of the practical and theoretical consequences of these hypotheses will be postponed till Chapter 13.

Finally, it is worth while quoting from a paper by Freud on the technique of psycho-analysis, which was published in 1913:

> 'One must distrust all prospective patients who want to make a delay before beginning their treatment. Experience shows that when the time agreed upon has arrived they fail to put in an appearance, even though the motive for the delay . . . seems to the uninitiated to be above suspicion.'

This is perhaps the earliest recorded statement about the relation between motivation and prognosis. Further evidence will be put forward later to illustrate apparent confirmation in our work of principles long accepted in psycho-analysis.

CHAPTER 10

The General Characteristics of these Therapies with Special Reference to Technique

THE ECOLOGICAL VIEW

As has already been emphasized (pp. 41 and 179 above), this whole research can be regarded as a natural experiment on the interaction between a population of patients on the one hand, and a number of psycho-analysts working in a group on the other, in which the latter's training, way of working, and interrelations almost certainly played a major part. This interaction is highly relevant to many aspects of our work—for instance, it was shown on p. 179 above to have had an all-important effect upon the characteristics of the patients under study; and on p. 274 below it will form an important step in the interpretation of some of the evidence and in drawing the whole work together. For present purposes this point of view will be used to shed light not only on the characteristics of these therapies, but also on some of the problems which are raised by the history of psycho-analysis and which have already been considered in Chapter 2.

RAPID AND INEVITABLE DEVELOPMENT OF TRANSFERENCE

One of the first important lessons that we learned was that in certain cases it is quite impossible to avoid the development of powerful transference feelings—even, sometimes, in the very earliest stage of the patient's contact with the clinical situation. The clearest example of this is a patient (the Student Nurse) not included in the present series because she was reported to the Workshop in retrospect and largely from memory:

> This hysterical girl of 19, at interview and in two subsequent sessions, was both apprehensive and uncooperative, forestalling questions by trying to interview the therapist. One of the themes

199

of her questions was what psychiatrists did to patients. At one point in session 2 she said 'This interview is quite different from what I expected when I talked to my friends about it', and she seemed to be implying that she consented to come only in order to be able to tell her friends what a psychiatric interview was like. The therapist managed to control his rising temper, and in the next session finally interpreted that she had been trying to make him angry, with which she at once agreed. He then suggested that perhaps she did something similar to her boy friend—tried to tantalize him so that he would lose his temper with her. She said yes. She said that she had had all sorts of phantasies about the interview—that the psychiatrist would have strange machines and peculiar tests and do horrible things to her. The therapist did not openly relate this to sexuality, but there followed a discussion of her conflict about whether or not to have intercourse with her boy friend. The tense situation was completely resolved, and she eventually said that she thought she had been understood and did not need to come any more.

This example has been chosen because it provides clear evidence that the patient had developed a definite transference (almost certainly connected with her anxieties about sex) in phantasy *before ever she arrived at the clinic*; and thus that even if the interviewer's behaviour may in some way have intensified this transference, nothing in his behaviour could possibly have brought it on in the first place.

Although there was no case as striking as this in the series under study here, there were many examples of patients whose transference feelings developed very early (see, for instance, the Lighterman), including some whose problems were such as to be activated almost automatically by the clinical situation:

The Pilot's Wife. The interviewer's written report opens as follows: 'Apparently when she arrived . . . and heard that she was going to see a man doctor she flatly refused . . . but when told that she would have to wait a fortnight before an appointment could be made with a woman psychiatrist . . . she eventually came up to see me.'

Almost the whole of the first half of therapy was taken up with her need to frustrate the male therapist, and with the link between this and her frigidity.

The Dog Lady. This patient, one of whose main problems was her intolerance of anger, tried to arrange her whole life so that people were nice and kind to her and she did not have to be angry. The interviewer, who knew that he would not be able to treat her himself, was deliberately rather distant and objective in order not to become too deeply involved with her. The third sentence of the therapist's written account of his first session with her reads: 'When I asked her why she felt like this she very quickly began talking about her interview with Dr. X. She said that she felt that he was cold. She had to have people be especially nice to her and this niceness must of course be sincere. . . .'

This rapid and inevitable development of transference is something that is little discussed in the literature, and that we therefore had to discover for ourselves. It is implied in some of Alexander and French's case histories (e.g. Case B, already quoted); but, so far as I know, is openly discussed only by Vosburg (op. cit. 1958) in his study of the case notes of therapies conducted by psychiatric residents:

'In the first three hours, an initial history of the patient is taken, and the patient invariably reacts to his disclosures with strong feelings. . . . Over the next several interviews . . . the material is distinguished from the opening hours . . . by the fact that the physician tends to become the object of the patient's feelings.'

This study of Vosburg's confirms several of our own observations (e.g. those on motivation already discussed, pp. 196–7), and Vosburg's whole idea of making a study of case histories will be used to introduce a study of my own in Chapter 12.

INEVITABLE DEVELOPMENT OF TRANSFERENCE INTERPRETATIONS

One of the clearest examples of the powerful forces developed on both sides by the interaction between these patients and the Workshop was the way in which our original fear of making transference interpretations (particularly prominent in myself) was ignored almost as soon as the work was started. Thus, parallel with the inevitability of transference in the patients was the inevitability of transference *interpretation* by the therapists. This may be illustrated by the following quotations from the Storm Lady:

Discussion after initial interview:

Malan: 'The moment the transference gets more important than reality you have "had it". If you can do anything before that point you may get there.'

201

Discussion after session 3:
(Therapist describes his technique of interpreting the associations to Rorschach cards.)

> *Therapist*: 'It arose from our discussion . . . that if one got involved in transference with this woman it would become a long-term case . . . when I interpret the material to her I interpret it in relation to the card and not at all to me.'

(Therapist now reports the material of sessions 2 and 3.)

> *Malan*: 'Because you deliberately were unable to talk about the transference there was very little in the session. . . .'
>
> *Mrs. Balint*: 'I cannot see how you can get on without making a transference interpretation.'

The result of this discussion was that of twenty-four interpretations recorded in the next session, eight referred to the transference; and one of these was that the patient felt as if she had been raped by the therapist, to which there was a dramatic positive response.

The important transference interpretation in session 3 of the Lighterman was the result of a similar discussion (see Assessment and Therapy Form, p. 96 above).

In fact, transference interpretations occur in all of the case histories in the present study with the exception of that of the Hypertensive Housewife. In a number of cases, of which the Railway Solicitor, the Lighterman, the Unsuccessful Accountant, and the Pilot's Wife are examples, the transference first caused a serious obstacle to therapeutic work which could only be—or, at any rate, could be—removed by interpretation; and then played a major part in interpretations throughout much of the rest of therapy. In these cases it is difficult to see how therapy without transference interpretation could have ended in any way other than permanent deadlock. It would be most interesting to know how this observation fits in with the statement of Rogers (see p. 32 above)—which I do not disbelieve—that in client-centred therapy the transference rarely causes any difficulty.

DISTURBING INTERPRETATIONS

The discovery (made very early in this work) that interpretation of the transference apparently did no harm, and might indeed form one of the major therapeutic factors, led to our feeling free to use a technique containing almost all the elements (except passivity) in which we had been trained as psycho-analysts, and very little else; and this in turn led to an ever more radical quality in therapy and in the hypotheses made about it.

We soon found, for instance, that any qualms we may have had about giving apparently disturbing interpretations were largely groundless. This does not mean that we practised a sort of 'wild analysis', flinging guesses about the patient's psychopathology in his face at the first opportunity, so to speak. On the contrary, we always first prepared the ground well by partial interpretations, gauging in this way not only what interpretations were correct but how much the patient could bear. Thus, when the time came, these disturbing interpretations could be made without fear or circumlocution, and almost always with the result not of increasing the patient's anxiety but of giving relief. When I was a casualty officer I once gave an ill-considered interpretation about death wishes to a patient in the first interview, and I now carry with me the chastening and guilt-laden memory of how he returned a few days later in a frankly psychotic state. Similarly, Alexander and French (op. cit. 1946) quote a case of a young man (Case T) who, after receiving interpretations about an Oedipal dream in the second session, developed paranoid delusions—and the situation was saved only by a very skilful intervention by the therapist in session 3. There were no such unfortunate results in the present work—even with the Paranoid Engineer there could be open talk about his wanting to burn his penis with a red-hot iron, or cause his father to be electrocuted. At the end of the session in which these themes were discussed the patient said that 'he felt we had made more progress . . . than in the ten previous sessions'.

In fact, what usually happened was that patient and therapist advanced together towards this kind of disturbing material, each in turn taking a step a little beyond the point already reached by the other, so that the final interpretation was in a sense clearly demanded by the patient and almost inevitable. This process is very important and is worth illustrating in some detail. The case chosen is again that of the Storm Lady:

> The essential interpretation towards which therapist and patient worked together was that the storm phobia represented her fear of her own wish to submit to violent sexuality. The first step towards this was made in the initial interview, when the therapist saved a difficult situation by interpreting that the storm represented 'powerful primitive natural forces' that she was afraid would overwhelm her. She said that that was in fact how she felt and immediately went on to speak of finding her

father unconscious and 'looking like an ape' after an accident.

In session 2 this subject was not touched on. In session 3 preliminary interpretations along the same lines led to her speaking of the Rotor at a fun fair, and the way that 'people are pushed against it by centrifugal force and are flung back with the arms splayed out; they look quite powerless'. The therapist interpreted that this description could be that of a person in 'an attitude of complete sexual submission'; and later related this to 'her fear of submitting to the overpowering dominant man'. There followed a discussion, without much intense communication, of the development of her sexual feelings when she was a girl.

In session 4, however, the patient had an outburst of guilt and shame about childhood masturbation, and the therapist's notes continue: [Therapist] 'You feel that I have forcefully broken down your façade and that the terrible shameful side of yourself is revealed.' [Patient] 'I think you can now see the real me.' (Report continues): 'I [therapist] say that the breaking down of the façade has something in common with a rape situation, which is what unconsciously she feels our present relationship to be—that she had been completely overcome by some very powerful force to which she can only submit with utter degradation.' [Patient] 'I just had to tell you, but I certainly felt as if I was giving in to you. *I noticed at the time that it was raining outside, and it occurred to me that if I were to see lightning which is a thing I fear most of all it would not matter the slightest bit to me—I would not be afraid.*' (My italics.)

This illustrates very clearly how a well-judged interpretation of disturbing material may result not in disturbance but in relief. The element missing from these interpretations, however, was the patient's sexual feelings about her father, which was approached in this session but never quite reached until much later in therapy, and was then ineffective.

INTERPRETATION OF THE INFANTILE ROOTS OF NEUROSIS
This ability to give disturbing interpretations without fear leads at once to the question of whether it is necessary or advisable to explore the infantile roots of neurosis in brief psychotherapy. Much evidence on this question will be put forward later (see pp. 248–60). Here nothing more will be said than that these infantile roots were frequently—though not always—explored, and that the response to this, and particularly to interpretations linking the transference situation to the childhood relation with

parents, was frequently clear and sometimes dramatic. This may be illustrated by the following quotations from the case notes (the most dramatic examples are unfortunately too complex to be suitable for quotation):

The first is concerned with the Oedipal situation in a woman. Here the male therapist was interpreted as the mother in the transference:

The Falling Social Worker (*session ?30*). 'In today's interview I tried to explore more deeply her reaction to having been sent away to hospital,[1] and the meaning in the difference in the atmosphere of the sessions since her return, and what emerged is as follows.

She was really much more angry than she has allowed me to find out so far about my apparent indifference on her return; she feels in fact that I have quite changed in my behaviour towards her, and that my taking up with her the question of a leaving date and so on was a confirmation of this indifference. This led to the whole question of the distance between us, and her relationship to her mother who was distant and indifferent to her; and what is more significant is that mother's indifference and distance are a thing which infuriates her. Mother won't share experiences with her, mother won't get excited about things the way she does, and this of course in a way seems to mean that mother condemns her excitement about these things.

I interpreted the guilt about the revenge on mother, that in fact the patient getting excited now shows mother that she can do things which mother can't do, whereas of course in childhood the situation was the reverse; and she went on to admit that this was true, and that she is with reading, for instance, always showing mother that she gets more out of things than mother does, and this led on to her saying that perhaps as a child she really wanted to make mother jealous by the excitement of her relationship with her father. . . .'

The second is concerned with a conflict over childhood dependence. Here also the male therapist was interpreted as the mother in the transference:

The Lighterman (*session 15*). 'After about half an hour he began to talk about his fear of the river, and the theme which emerged was how he hated the river and blamed it for a lot of his trouble because in his job one had to wait around so much and never knew when one would be given a job or what one would have to do next.

[1] The patient had been ill.

205

I felt he was asking me for interpretation, and I interpreted this first in his relation to his mother and having to wait for her to look after him or feed him, and then in relation to myself, that I had kept him waiting for two months before seeing him. He denied this vigorously and then told me that he had had a row today with a shop to which he had given a specimen hinge to copy, and which had given him the wrong hinge back. I showed him how this might apply to me and suggested that he felt he wanted to criticize me for not getting him well quickly enough. He again denied this but immediately spoke of a doctor whom he had recently gone to and who had treated him much better than his usual GP. He had a moment of thought-blocking in which he said that he felt that there was some criticism of me in his mind but he could not remember what it was. Eventually I brought out a little criticism about the way in which I had let him go off last time with the thought that there was an impulse to suicide in him and without reassuring him.'

At one point in these therapies, interpretations became as 'deep' as in the following example:

The Articled Accountant (*session 17*). 'I came to the conclusion that I would have to make a vigorous attempt to interpret the depression in two-person terms. For some reason it came to me that the language I should use was "being angry with someone that he loved". . . . I went on to translate this into inside-outside terms, saying that it was as if he went through the world taking good experiences into himself from his parents, from me, from everybody else, but that now that he had to think about leaving his parents and me it was as if he was so angry that he was trying to destroy what good things we had given to him, which he felt to be inside himself, and thus it became almost physical and he felt he had killed something inside himself. . . .'
(Two paragraphs later):
'Shortly after this he said, "I have just remembered something". He went on to say that all through his life he had always accepted the inevitable; for instance, when he left school he had accepted that he had to go to the university, but when the university came near he had not really looked forward to it. I immediately said that this applied to all sorts of parallel situations: school to university was the same as university to world or home to world or this clinic to world, and I repeated that perhaps he was so angry at having school or mother or my care taken away from him that he really wanted to smash up inside himself all the good

things which he had taken from us. Shortly after this he said that he used to go through life and meet people thinking that he was quite easy-going and although his feelings did not seem to be very deep . . . he had come to realize they were quite violent.'

It should be noted that some evidence will be presented in the next chapter that if a therapist gives this kind of interpretation to *deeply* depressive patients he may well find himself involved in a therapy which can no longer be described as 'brief'.

Apart from the special situation mentioned in the previous paragraph, however, there was no evidence that interpretations of the infantile roots of neurosis, at any rate when given by these particular therapists to these particular patients, either did the patient harm or caused an unmanageable increase in the length of therapy. This conclusion is in marked contrast to the implied views of a number of conservative authors already quoted in Chapter 3.

NEGATIVE TRANSFERENCE: TERMINATION

The reader may have noted that all three of the passages just quoted refer to *negative* transference, and moreover to a particular aspect of this, namely anger at *termination* or the loss of the therapist's care for other reasons. It was over the question of negative transference that our radical approach reached its climax. This came about over a particular patient, the Draper's Assistant, in the following way:

The patient, whose complaint was non-consummation of marriage, was originally thought to have provided one of our most striking successes. She had reported at the end of therapy that she had had intercourse several times, and later that she and her husband were thinking of starting a family. When she was seen for follow-up, two years later, she admitted under pressure that she had not really had intercourse at all.

The report of this in the Workshop caused a good deal of consternation; but there eventually emerged the suggestion that this girl's real problem was her need to frustrate people, which she expressed towards her husband by refusing intercourse, and towards the therapist by pretending to an improvement which had not really occurred at all. It was suggested that, since this problem had never been brought into the open in the transference, it was not surprising that therapy had been a failure. This led to the hypothesis that an essential part of almost every therapy was for the patient to pass through and learn to tolerate his negative feelings towards the therapist, since only in this way could he learn to tolerate these feelings in relation to people outside. Moreover, the situation in which the patient was most likely to experience negative feelings was over the withdrawal of the therapist's care at termination. If these feelings were not brought into the open and worked through, and the relation with the therapist remained idealized, there was a very real danger that the patient might spoil the therapeutic result in order to spite the therapist:

Quotation from summary of Workshop discussion: 'Mrs. Balint makes the point that . . . during the therapy the therapist must become a bad figure, accepted as such and tolerated by the patient; otherwise only idealization can occur.'

The application of this principle to a particular patient may be illustrated by a quotation from a much later discussion:

Main (T. F.): 'I feel strongly about this—unless the conditions of parting can allow the man's rage at termination to come into the open, the therapy is in danger.'

This attitude to the negative transference marked the crystallization of a stage in the development of our ideas corresponding to that introduced into psycho-analysis by Ferenczi and Rank (op. cit.), and more recently re-emphasized in Alexander and French's concept of the 'corrective emotional experience': that the experience of the old problems in the relation with the therapist —but with a new ending—is the most important single factor in therapy.

DIFFERENCES FROM ANALYSIS

Since the whole emphasis of the preceding pages has been on the similarities between our technique and that of psycho-analysis, the question may well be asked how it was that most of these therapies did not in the end become like analysis. The answer we would probably give to this is that our therapies differed from analysis in three main ways: (i) they had a limited aim; (ii) the patient was made to understand from the beginning that the number of sessions would be limited; and (iii) the technique was 'focal'.

The concept of limited aim is one which is common to most forms of brief psychotherapy and need not be considered at length. One point is worth noting, however: that, although limited aims were sometimes stated in terms of *therapeutic results*, what was almost invariably practised was a limited aim in terms of *working through briefly a given aspect of psychopathology* and, in effect, seeing what result would follow. This has advantages, because the therapeutic result may be greater than could possibly be expected. With the Biologist the original aim was to relieve his eating phobia; what happened in fact was that the therapist made as his aim the brief working through of passive homosexuality; and the therapeutic result included not only the relief of the eating phobia, but also an improvement in his potency and in his relation with his wife.

The technique that we eventually developed for conveying the limitations of therapy to the patient was to put to him, at the beginning, some such statement as the following: 'My idea is to go ahead with treatment, once a week, for a few months and see where we can get. At the end of that time we will review the situation, but if it looks as if you need more you will be transferred to a longer form of treatment. If we feel we have got far enough, then I will stop seeing you *regularly*. This does not mean that you will necessarily stop seeing me altogether—you can ask to come back at any time for further occasional sessions if you feel you need further help.'

Sometimes the task of limiting therapy was made easier by the fact that the patient himself had only a limited time available (e.g. the Biologist). The more difficult question of definite time limits set in advance by the therapist was the subject of some uneasiness at first. In fact this technique was used with success in the Falling Social Worker (in-patient, forty sessions) in the present series of cases, and in several later cases (out-patients, sixteen to twenty sessions) not included in the present study. It was a failure in the Storm Lady, where the therapist's original aim was to see her for ten sessions, one for each Rorschach card; and, with a quite unrealistic limit of eight sessions set by the therapist's departure from the clinic, in the Paranoid Engineer. The setting of an exact time limit in advance does not—as might easily be expected—seem to make the work impossible; but on the contrary gives the treatment a definite 'beginning, a middle, and an end' (Phillips and Johnston, op. cit. 1954), and seems to facilitate the therapist's task of dealing with feelings about termination. Since this technique was little used in the present series of patients, however, it will not be considered further.

Similarly, though the offer of further sessions in case of need may possibly have played a part in maintaining patients after termination, the present series of patients offers little evidence about this, and it also will not be considered further.

The 'focal' technique, on the other hand, is a subject in itself, and will be considered next.

THE 'FOCAL' TECHNIQUE: 'FOCAL THERAPY'

This technique can perhaps be described in the following way: the therapist keeps in his mind an aim or 'focus', which should ideally be formulated in terms of an essential interpretation on which therapy is to be based. He pursues this focus single-mindedly: he guides the patient towards it by partial interpretations, selective attention, and selective neglect; if the material admits of more than one interpretation he always chooses that which is consonant with the focus; and he refuses to be diverted by material apparently irrelevant to the focus, however tempting this may be.

Obviously this technique is based on the principles of *activity* and *planning* adopted by many authors, and on the 'skilful neglect' mentioned by Pumpian-Mindlin, and it has much in common with the aims—though not the methods—of the 'associative anamnesis' of Deutsch. It is a deliberate attempt to overcome several of the lengthening factors: passivity, the willingness to follow where the patient leads, and—by keeping therapy simple—over-determination.

Obviously, too, it depends entirely on a successful interaction between patient and therapist, which—by analogy with an idea expressed in Balint's book (1957)—may be described thus: (a) the patient offers material, which (b) enables the therapist to formulate a focus, which (c) the therapist offers to the patient, which (d) the patient in turn accepts and works with.

This preliminary mutual offering can often be seen quite clearly in the initial interview and one or two subsequent sessions, resulting finally in the *crystallization* of a focus on which most of the rest of therapy is based. Moreover, since the therapists in the present work were continually reporting back to the Workshop and receiving criticism and advice, the other members of the Workshop—led by Balint's extensive experience—also played an important part in the interaction. This whole process may be illustrated by the case of the Biologist (although the word 'focus' had not yet been introduced, the principles were exactly the same):

This patient was originally seen by a non-Workshop psychiatrist, and then for a Rorschach by the psychologist (= therapist) who

210

took him on for treatment. It was noticed by both the interviewer and the psychologist that latent homosexuality seemed to be a problem for the patient, but no special emphasis was laid on this. The psychologist was more impressed by one of the Rorschach responses, which seemed to link up with an emotionally significant event in the patient's family history; and he felt that the patient's feelings about this might be an important focus in therapy. He also noticed in the Rorschach that mouths seemed to be important to the patient, and he felt that the eating phobia might be connected with fellatio phantasies and that these might form another focus.

In fact, in session 1 (and indeed in subsequent therapy) the patient brought hardly any material that seemed to connect with the event in his family history, and this focus was quickly forgotten. It was discovered later that the therapist had understood the details wrongly and that the event was likely to have been much less emotionally significant than had been originally supposed. Similarly, two loaded questions by the therapist designed to lead towards fellatio, met with no response, e.g.: 'I then took a chance, and said "Perhaps phantasies in which the mouth occurs are particularly exciting?" This had no apparent meaning to him, and he said, "I'm not with you there".'

On the other hand, what the patient's material did concern was, almost entirely, his *relation with men*. Thus he opened session 1 by telling how the first attack of his phobia had occurred when he was having a meal in the train with his boss. The therapist made a number of partial interpretations: (i) that perhaps his feelings about men in authority would be important; (ii) that in relation to this type of man he had difficulty in coping with his aggressive feelings; (iii) that rivalry seemed to be important. This last interpretation led to an account by the patient of how he could not serve at tennis when playing with his father-in-law because his forearm 'went like india-rubber'. The therapist, translating the symbolism, immediately said 'I think this leads us to . . . your anxieties about impotence', to which the patient, surprised, at once admitted. The therapist then made a general comment saying that he seemed to have problems of aggression with men and, since this paralysis of his forearm occurred in his relation with a man, perhaps of homosexuality also. Again the patient looked surprised, admitted that homosexual feelings were returning, and went on to speak of his compulsive phantasies.

211

The exploratory nature of this interview was in fact criticized in the Workshop—especially by Balint, who advocated that the therapist should have given a number of somewhat 'wild' interpretations at once: that he should have interpreted the sexual meaning of 'serve' and suggested that the patient felt he could not 'serve' a man but wanted to be 'served' by him; and that eating in public is 'accepting that he is pregnant and showing he is pregnant by being sick'. He suggested that the therapist had concentrated on aggression rather than on passive homosexuality because 'aggression' is an easier word to use than 'love'.

From all these suggested interpretations the general focus of the patient's relations with men, with special reference to passive homosexuality, crystallized for both patient and therapist during the next two sessions, and was maintained with little deviation for the rest of therapy. The main theme of every session, and of the great majority of individual interpretations, was related to this focus. As already described, the eating phobia was apparently relieved by the recall of a homosexual incident at school which had later become associated with a meal table.

Selective neglect may be illustrated by the case of the Lighterman:

The focus which crystallized in session 3 and became further clarified in session 5 was the patient's childhood conflict over his feelings for his mother—a mixture of intense anger and guilt. This focus, first guilt and then anger, was pursued fairly single-mindedly by patient and therapist until session 14, when the patient opened up the question of his *fears of suicide*. Now this problem could certainly be related to the main focus, but the therapist felt that any attempt to include it in the focus would lead into water much too deep for brief therapy. He therefore, during this single session, interpreted all aspects of the problem that seemed appropriate; but when the patient (who by now was spacing his own sessions) said that if the therapist allowed him to stay away for two months he would feel reassured that the therapist was not worried that he would in fact commit suicide, the therapist accepted this with a mixture of apprehension and relief. The gap was sufficient for the patient to bury his suicidal feelings; and, though mentioned, they did not cause any further difficulty during the rest of therapy.

This selective neglect by allowing a gap in therapy is a technical device borrowed from Alexander and French.

It is clearly true that the possibility of using a highly 'focal' technique depends on the patient as well as on the therapist; and since therapy was relatively 'focal' in the majority of these patients, it seems that 'focality' (so to speak) was one of the criteria on which patients were selected. 'Focality' may be defined as the ability of patient and therapist together to find a focus quickly which is acceptable to both of them. In other words, an important selection criterion (which has recently been especially advocated by Balint) may be that a workable focus should crystallize within the first few sessions. Since these earlier patients were so heavily selected in favour of this criterion, its value cannot, unfortunately, be studied here.

As our work has developed, an increasing emphasis has been laid on the 'focal' aspect of technique, until finally our particular form of brief psychotherapy has come to be known as Focal Therapy.

DRAMATIC THERAPY; TRAUMATIC MEMORIES

There are two final characteristics of these therapies which are of great interest: (i) dramatic responses to interpretation, and (ii) the recall of traumatic memories, or—perhaps more correctly— 'cover memories'. The first has already been illustrated sufficiently in the Assessment and Therapy Forms and elsewhere (e.g. the Storm Lady, p. 204). The traumatic memories are listed below:

The Lighterman:	the accident to the little girl.
The Biologist:	the mention of his homosexual episode at a meal table.
The Paranoid Engineer:	the incident in which he had (so he said) been homosexually assaulted as a child.

Now it is also true that, proportionately, these dramatic responses to interpretation occurred far more frequently in the six cases treated in the first year than in the thirteen treated in the second. Moreover, all three of the traumatic memories listed above occurred in the first year. The interest of this observation lies in the comparison with the early analyses, which were also dramatic, and in which the unearthing of traumatic memories was felt to be the main work of therapy. It will be remembered that Balint and several other authors have suggested that the factor leading to this dramatic quality in therapy is the intense interaction

213

engendered by the therapist's enthusiasm. Our work thus provides some slight circumstantial evidence in favour of this view, because there is little doubt that during the first year of our work our enthusiasm was highest, and that during the second year it waned.

There is also some circumstantial evidence that—just as, apparently, with the early analyses—this high enthusiasm has a favourable effect on therapeutic *results*. In four and a half years of work, during which about fifty patients have been treated by a total of eleven therapists, the most successful cases are to be found not among those treated by any particular therapist, but much more obviously among the *first and second cases treated for the Workshop* by each of a number of different therapists. (Of the eight results that probably qualify for a score of 3, four are provided by first cases, two by second cases, and only two by the remainder—the proportion of scores of 3 among first and second cases together being about 30 per cent as against about 7 per cent for the remainder. With such small numbers this is of course quite without statistical significance.)

This interesting observation, which is as yet of course not properly documented, suggests the possibility that the emotional conditions within the therapist—always known to be important—may be even more important than has yet been realized, and may sometimes make the whole difference between an interminable failure and a quick success. This factor may also partly account for the great divergence in views to be found in the literature—since if conditions within the therapists are not reproducible, therapeutic results may not be reproducible either. The authors with the most radical views about results may be those who have been fortunate enough to undertake therapy—for a time at any rate—under conditions likely to lead to the maximum enthusiasm. This entirely 'non-specific' factor may indeed sometimes override the importance of technique itself (cf. Strupp, 1960, pp. 318ff.), and may explain why such widely differing techniques seem to be capable of producing comparable therapeutic results.

CHAPTER 11

The Relation between Transference Interpretation and Outcome: Clinical Approach

INTRODUCTION

It will be remembered that we, in common with a number of conservative authors, originally held the view that for various reasons transference interpretations would be dangerous in brief psychotherapy—that they themselves would intensify transference, or cause the transference to become more primitive, or increase dependence, or hasten the onset of the transference neurosis—in any case, that they would tend to make termination difficult and lead in some way or other to an unfavourable outcome; and that in fact our views, based on clinical impression, became ever more radical, until ultimately the hypothesis was made that interpretation of the negative transference was an essential factor in therapy. The examination of the evidence relevant to these and similar hypotheses will occupy a large part of the remainder of this book, and will lead far afield, through problems of methodology, follow-up, and selection criteria, finally to an overall view of the whole nature of this kind of therapy and the place which it holds in the history of psychoanalytic technique.

CLINICAL EVIDENCE

Now, with the exception of the Hypertensive Housewife, transference interpretations were made in all these therapies; and there was a clear response to these *at some time* in all cases except those of Tom and the Student's Wife (the case of the Draper's Assistant is equivocal, see below). Thus, once more, we are dealing with therapies concentrated at the 'upper' end of a scale, this time the scale of 'transference orientation'. If the relation between transference orientation and outcome is to be studied, therefore, some way must be found either of introducing a quantitative element

215

TABLE 11 RATIONALE FOR SCORING 'TRANSFERENCE ORIENTATION' ON A 4-POINT SCALE

Patient	Score	Rationale
Biologist	1	The main work was done outside the transference, leading to the dramatic breakthrough in session 6. Transference was probably important in session 3 (resistance interpretation); perhaps in session 8. Little response to interpretations about termination.
Lighterman	2	He is judged to score 2 on the grounds that, although there was intense transference work at the beginning and end of therapy, there was a long period of direct work on the relation with his mother in the middle, in which the transference was ignored.
Neurasthenic's Husband	3	In early sessions transference and non-transference work seem to have been of about equal importance. No marked response at any time, but steady progress. The really intense moment of therapy was concerned with transference over termination (sessions 13 and 14).
Falling Social Worker	3	The main work of therapy seems to have been that on the dependent sexual transference to the present and previous therapists. As with the Neurasthenic's Husband, however, this was interspersed with much work on feelings about parents.
Railway Solicitor	3	Transference interpretations concerned with the main focus of anxieties about relations with men were the main theme of almost every session from the very beginning. There was a middle period in which transference interpretations became less important, but response here was probably not clear (this part of therapy is not recorded). Transference interpretations again became important as termination approached.
Girl with the Dreams	2	Therapy was divided into two halves: 8 sessions of mainly transference work; then 10 sessions of mainly non-transference work. It is possible that the score should be 3 since responses were more clear-cut in the second half.

Case	Score	Notes
Civil Servant	3	The main focus of sessions 3–8 seems to have been inability to disagree with the therapist, who was interpreted as the father in the transference. Work on the direct relation with the father was also done. In sessions 9–12 there was both work on the transference to the therapist as a woman and non-transference work on sexual anxieties.
Surgeon's Daughter	2	The main focus was inability to be angry or press her claims. The therapist did about equal amounts of work on this in relation to the patient's fiancé and in the transference.
Unsuccessful Accountant	3	The tension in the transference was the main focus in session 6 in which the patient himself interpreted this as being due to homosexual feelings.
Draper's Assistant	?3	Very difficult to judge. If the attempted intercourse is regarded as a response to the one important transference interpretation, then the score of 3 is certain; if, on the other hand, this was just a response to pressure from therapist and husband, the appropriate score is 0.
Storm Lady	1	Therapist did his best to concentrate on non-transference work. Important transference interpretations were isolated.
Tom	0	Practically all the work was outside the transference. Only one transference interpretation is recorded, to which the response was not clear.
Hypertensive Housewife	0	Therapist's report at discussion: 'What I have tried to do is not to give her any transference interpretations.' In fact, hardly any interpretations which can really be classed as referring to the transference are recorded.
Pilot's Wife	3	There is no question that practically the whole of the work was carried out through the transference.

Table 11—*continued*

Patient	Score	Rationale
Student Thief	1	The therapist's main efforts were directed outside the transference in sessions 1–8 and brought clear response. There was a single important transference interpretation, to which there was also a clear response, in session 9.
Paranoid Engineer	3	The breakthrough in session 4 was apparently a transference experience and immediately followed a transference interpretation. The later intense session (10) was mainly outside the transference but was related to the transference at the end. (Possibly the score should be 2.)
Violet's Mother	1	The therapist's main efforts were directed outside the transference for the first 10 sessions, with some response. The last sessions were mainly concerned with termination and also brought some response. Perhaps the score should be 2.
Articled Accountant	2	Therapy was divided into two halves: 13 sessions of non-transference work leading to apparent improvement; 14 sessions mainly concerned with termination, leading to the sudden lifting of depression.
Student's Wife	0	No effective transference work. Breakthrough in session 6 was entirely outside the transference.

into the judgements, or of breaking transference down into different categories and studying each of these qualitatively in isolation. Both approaches will be used.

Transference Interpretation in General

A way of introducing a quantitative element is to make a judgement of the *relative 'importance'* of transference and non-transference work in each therapy. If circular arguments are to be avoided this word 'importance' needs to be carefully defined:

The 'importance' of a given kind of interpretative work is judged to have been high:

1. quantitatively, if many such interpretations were made and either there was ultimately a clear response, or else the patient was clearly working with them step by step;
2. qualitatively, if there was a very marked response to one or a few isolated interpretations.

With these criteria, I have judged 'transference orientation' on the four-point scale below:

Score 3: Transference work more important than non-transference.

Score 2: Transference and non-transference work of equal importance.

Score 1: Transference used but less important than non-transference.

Score 0: Transference work of hardly any importance at all.

These judgements were made about two years ago, long before I had carried out the studies to be presented in Chapter 12, and I am not sure that I would agree with all of them now. Nevertheless—since this may well be due to contamination with my own later conclusions—I present them entirely unchanged, and with my notes written down at the time no more than somewhat edited.

The rationale for the scores is shown in *Table 11*, and the scores in relation to outcome in *Table 12*.

Inspection of *Table 12* will show: (i) that the hypothesis that a high transference orientation is *harmful* is strongly contradicted; (ii) that, on the contrary, the hypothesis that a high transference orientation is (statistically) a *necessary condition* to success is supported by the evidence (the only case that contradicts the hypothesis is the Biologist); but (iii) that the hypothesis of *parallel variation* is less certainly supported—there being a number of less

TABLE 12 'TRANSFERENCE ORIENTATION'
IN RELATION TO OUTCOME

Patient	Score for outcome	Score for 'transference orientation'
Biologist	3	1
Lighterman	3	2
Neurasthenic's Husband	3	3
Falling Social Worker	3	3
Railway Solicitor	3	3
Girl with the Dreams	2	2
Civil Servant	1	3
Surgeon's Daughter	1	2
Unsuccessful Accountant	1	3
Draper's Assistant	0	?3
Storm Lady	0	1
Tom	0	0
Hypertensive Housewife	0	0
Pilot's Wife	0	3
Student Thief	0	1
Paranoid Engineer	0	3
Violet's Mother	0	1
Articled Accountant	0	2
Student's Wife	0	0

successful therapies with a high transference orientation. If the last hypothesis is given the best possible chance, i.e. if the doubtful case that contradicts the hypothesis—the Draper's Assistant—is omitted, τ_b hovers on the brink of the 5 per cent level of 'significance' ($\tau_b = +0.41$, $p = 0.051$). If the Draper's Assistant is included, $\tau_b = +0.34$ and p becomes 0.1—a clear example of how sensitive these correlations are to single changes of judgement, and therefore how little reliance can be placed upon any one of them in isolation.

Negative Transference

If we now proceed to the second kind of approach, that of breaking down the transference into subdivisions, we may first consider the 'hypothesis of the necessary condition' relating to negative transference. The formal statement of this is:

A necessary condition to success is that interpretation of the negative transference should be 'important' at some stage in therapy.

The evidence, with negative transference scored on a three-point scale, is shown in *Table 13*.

As it stands, this table is quite striking. In clinical terms, *all* cases that give a score for outcome higher than 0 contained some successful work on negative transference, whereas six out of ten cases that score 0 for outcome contain either no response to interpretation of negative transference or even no recorded interpretation of negative transference at all. If both the scales are made dichotomous (a score of 0 on the one hand, and more than 0 on the other) and set out on a 2×2 contingency table, the distribution is as below:

	Negative transference	
Outcome	2 or 1	0
3, 2, or 1	9	0
0	4	6

Since cases in the bottom left-hand corner are irrelevant to a hypothesis of this kind, there are no cases in this series that contradict the hypothesis at all.

221

TABLE 13 NEGATIVE TRANSFERENCE
IN RELATION TO OUTCOME

Patient	Score for outcome	Score for negative trans- ference	Rationale
Biologist	3	1	Session 8: argument with therapist, with partial response to interpretation of negative feelings.
Lighterman	3	2	Session 11: criticism of therapist for not looking after him properly finally brought out. Session 17: marked response to interpretation about anger over therapist's holiday.
Neurasthenic's Husband	3	2	Marked response to interpretations about denigration of therapist and father as a defence against admitting a need for them.
Falling Social Worker	3	2	Session 30: therapist brings out clear anger over his indifference.
Railway Solicitor	3	1	Rivalry, fear of retaliation (not really 'negative'), dealt with in early part of therapy. Hostility over termination interpreted in later part, but no clear response.
Girl with the Dreams	2	1 (?2)	Sessions 12, 15: interpretation about wish to kill therapist off, no clear response. Session 18: clear dream about therapist as jealous mother.

Table 13—*continued*

Patient	Score for outcome	Score for negative trans- ference	Rationale
Civil Servant	1	2	Fear of disagreeing with therapist made into main focus, with final 'heated disagreement' in session 7.
Surgeon's Daughter	1	2	Session 9: partially successful interpretation about 'hateful feelings' for therapist. Session 16: clear anger with therapist brought out ('I get so annoyed when people don't understand me').
Unsuccessful Accountant	1	1	The tension between patient and therapist was interpreted as due to negative feelings in sessions 3, 4, 5, and 6. Patient eventually interpreted the tension as due to homosexual feelings, in which the quality of hostility was absent.
Draper's Assistant	0	0	The only interpretation approaching negative feelings was of the need to 'control' the therapist in session 5.
Storm Lady	0	0	Negative transference hardly touched on at any time.
Tom	0	0	The only hint of interpretation of negative feelings was of his symptoms as a way of forcing the therapist to take his decision for him.
Hypertensive Housewife	0	0	Hardly any transference interpretations at all.

Table 13—*continued*

Patient	Score for outcome	Score for negative trans-ference	Rationale
Pilot's Wife	0	2	Almost the whole of the early part of therapy devoted to interpreting the resentment against the therapist as a man and the need to frustrate him. Final response in session 11: 'I just have a hunch you might be right.'
Student Thief	0	2	Session 9: interpretation brings out open resentment about therapist's 'taking her for granted'.
Paranoid Engineer	0	0 (?1)	Session 10: patient feels he has had a 'fight' with therapist and proved himself a man. There was no quality of hostility in this fight.
Violet's Mother	0	2	Many interpretations of anger at termination (sessions 12, 13, 14). The only clear response was a counter-attack in session 12 ('Perhaps *you* feel guilty about termination'); and a reproach in session 13 that the therapist had 'held out a helping hand and then withdrawn it'.
Articled Accountant	0	2	Sessions 15–22: repeated attempts to bring out anger about termination, with final lifting of depression.
Student's Wife	0	0	Negative transference not interpreted at all.

The hypothesis of parallel variation, on the other hand, is not supported. This is largely because of the great importance of negative transference in a number of the less successful cases.

Transference at the Beginning and End of Therapy
Another way of subdividing transference interpretation is roughly (though not quite accurately) into:

1. transference interpretation on *entering* therapy, and
2. transference interpretation on *leaving* therapy.

To put this more accurately:

1. Whether or not transference interpretations become an 'important' (or 'major') issue early in therapy (within the first four sessions)—this to include the situation in which transference interpretations on a particular focus began to be made repeatedly within the first four sessions, though the actual response did not occur till later.

2. Whether or not interpretation of feelings about termination (grief and/or anger) became an 'important' issue at any point.

The rationale for scoring this on a rough four-point scale (Yes, Yes?, No?, and No) is shown in *Table 14*, and the scores in relation to outcome are shown in *Table 15*.

The material summarized in *Table 15* is interesting in that the answers to these two questions (i.e. whether transference on entering therapy and transference on leaving therapy were major issues)—and especially the answers to both questions taken together—constitute (so to speak) a far 'severer' test of these therapies than the answers to the similar questions about transference in general or negative transference alone. Thus, whereas the answers to the previous questions tended to make a distinction simply between 'successful' and 'unsuccessful' therapies, the answers to the present questions tend to go further, and to make a distinction between the 'more successful' and the 'less successful'. In fact, the only therapies that give a certainly positive answer to both of these present questions are one that scores 0 (the Articled Accountant) and the 'hard core' of those that score 3 (the Lighterman, the Neurasthenic's Husband, and the Falling Social Worker). Not only this, but the other two that score 3 are borderline cases giving a positive or doubtfully positive answer to the first question, and a doubtfully negative answer to the second.

A discussion of the exact meaning of this evidence will be

225

TABLE 14 WHETHER (1) EARLY TRANSFERENCE AND
(2) TRANSFERENCE OVER TERMINATION WERE 'IMPORTANT' ISSUES

Patient	Score for outcome	Transference a major issue in first four sessions	Transference over termination a major issue
Biologist	3	There was a single 'focal' transference resistance interpretation in session 3, to which there was a clear response and which resolved the resistance. **Yes?**	5 recorded interpretations (in session 10 only) about feelings of loss of therapist without clear response. **No?**
Lighterman	3	Session 3: dramatic response to interpretation of fear of being criticized by therapist, like his father, for being a nuisance to his mother. **Yes**	Sessions 11, 15, 17: much anxiety relieved by interpretations about patient's anger that the therapist had left him or was not available. **Yes**
Neurasthenic's Husband	3	Therapist began to interpret denigration of himself and patient's father in session 2. **Yes**	Interpretation that patient was trying to be independent as termination approached in order to avoid feelings of longing for a man (therapist or father) met with dramatic response. **Yes**
Falling Social Worker	3	Main focus of dependent sexual transference interpreted from session 1 onwards. **Yes**	Anger with therapist about his indifference when patient was ill clearly brought out (session 30). Grief at termination a major focus during last period of therapy. **Yes**
Railway Solicitor	3	Rivalry, etc. with therapist made main focus from session 1 onwards. **Yes**	Anger with therapist about termination interpreted with little response. **No?**

Girl with the Dreams	2	Hardly any transference work in first 4 sessions.	No	3 recorded interpretations about termination: 2 about grief (with open response); 1 about anger (with doubtful response). My own judgement that this was not a major issue.	No?
Civil Servant	1	Focus of inability to contradict therapist crystallized in session 3.	Yes	No recorded work on termination.	No
Surgeon's Daughter	1	Some transference interpretations with doubtful response in session 1, not in sessions 2–4.	No	Inability to be angry or to press her claims for further treatment made into an important focus with clear response in sessions 8, 9, and 11.	Yes
Unsuccessful Accountant	1	Transference focus of tension in sessions, related to patient's difficulties at interviews for jobs, crystallized in session 3.	Yes	No recorded work on termination.	No
Draper's Assistant	0	No recorded transference interpretations in first 4 sessions.	No	No recorded work on termination.	No
Storm Lady	0	'Focal' interpretation about feeling as if she had been raped by therapist produced a dramatic response in session 4.	Yes	One recorded interpretation about forthcoming break in therapy when she has her baby, with a clear response. But since it was implied that therapy would continue later, the question of termination was not really relevant.	No

Table 14—continued

Patient	Score for outcome	Transference a major issue in first four sessions		Transference over termination a major issue	
Tom	0	Only one transference interpretation recorded in the 4 sessions of therapy (session 3); doubtful response.	No	Work on termination not relevant—patient breaks off treatment.	—
Hypertensive Housewife	0	Hardly any transference work at any time.	No	Although no work on termination was recorded in the period of therapy under consideration, termination became a major issue in later therapy—which was still a failure. Therefore no score.	—
Pilot's Wife	0	The need to contradict everything the therapist said crystallized in sessions 3 and 4, and was made into the main focus of therapy from then on.	Yes	3 recorded interpretations about termination produced little response.	No
Student Thief	0	There were indications of disturbance in the transference in sessions 1 and 4. The first was resolved by the interpretation that asking her to come back for more therapy was like the matron pressing her to confess to the other thefts. This was a 'tactical' interpretation, not part of the main focus. The disturbance in session 4 was not interpreted.	No	No recorded work on termination.	No

Paranoid Engineer	0	Interpretation in session 4 that he did not feel masculine enough with the therapist led to dramatic re-enacting of being homosexually assaulted as a child.	Yes	No work on termination recorded; but since hardly any work on termination was done at the end of long-term therapy, and this still resulted in major gains: no score.	—
Violet's Mother	0	When patient said she wanted instruction from the therapist about how to handle her family, therapist interpreted that she was seeking from him the support which she had not received from her husband (session 4). This was interpreted also in later sessions, but never produced any clear response.	No?	Threat of termination brought relapse. The rest of therapy concerned with interpreting grief and anger over termination, with clear response on at least two occasions.	Yes
Articled Accountant	0	Session 4: clear response to the interpretation that patient wanted the therapist to tide him over the transition from being a boy to being a man.	Yes	Threat of termination brought depression. Anger and a sense of loss at termination were made into the main focus from session 15 to termination at session 27.	Yes
Student's Wife	0	Exploratory transference interpretations in session 1: (a) that she was afraid of being 'penetrated' by therapist's interpretations and (b) that she was asking for reassurance and permission, which was what she wanted from her mother, met with little response, and were not repeated in sessions 2-4.	No	A single recorded interpretation about a feeling of loss of the therapist met with little response.	No

TABLE 15 SUMMARY OF TABLE 14

Patient	Score for outcome	Transference a major issue in first 4 sessions	Transference over termination a major issue
Biologist	3	Yes?	No?
Lighterman	3	Yes	Yes
Neurasthenic's Husband	3	Yes	Yes
Falling Social Worker	3	Yes	Yes
Railway Solicitor	3	Yes	No?
Girl with the Dreams	2	No	No?
Civil Servant	1	Yes	No
Surgeon's Daughter	1	No	Yes
Unsuccessful Accountant	1	Yes	No
Draper's Assistant	0	No	No
Storm Lady	0	Yes	—
Tom	0	No	—
Hypertensive Housewife	0	No	—
Pilot's Wife	0	Yes	No
Student Thief	0	No	No
Paranoid Engineer	0	Yes	—
Violet's Mother	0	No?	Yes
Articled Accountant	0	Yes	Yes
Student's Wife	0	No	No

postponed till the last chapter. For the moment, all that will be said is that the evidence that transference interpretation—in one form or another—played a greater part in the successful than in the unsuccessful therapies can be seen to be very strong indeed.

TRANSFERENCE INTERPRETATION AND DEPENDENCE

The mere fact that important transference work seems on the whole to be associated with favourable outcome is enough to contradict the hypothesis that transference interpretations intensify dependence—or at least that they intensify it to the point at which termination becomes impossible without relapse. The detailed evidence on the relation between transference interpretations and dependence overwhelmingly confirms this conclusion:

1. Of the seven cases in which clinical judgement suggests that transference played the most important part (score of 3 for 'transference orientation'—omitting the Draper's Assistant):

   (a) in only one was there failure to terminate (the Paranoid Engineer);
   (b) in three there was no evidence for the development of dependence at all, and these were not among the most successful (the Civil Servant, the Unsuccessful Accountant, and the Pilot's Wife; scores 1, 1, and 0 for outcome respectively);
   (c) in the other three intense dependence did indeed develop, but (i) it could be handled by interpretation, (ii) it did not prove in the end a serious obstacle to termination, and (iii) these are three of the most successful cases of all (the 'hard core'—the Lighterman, the Neurasthenic's Husband, and the Falling Social Worker).

2. Of the two other cases in which the first stage of therapy ended in failure to terminate: (i) in the Hypertensive Housewife there were hardly any transference interpretations at all, and (ii) in the Storm Lady, apart from isolated intense transference sessions, the therapist did his best to concentrate on non-transference work throughout.

3. In the two cases in which threat of termination led to (i) immediate relapse, (ii) the revelation of a largely ignored dependent transference, and (iii) final failure, transference interpretations had hitherto played a very small part (the Articled Accountant, Violet's Mother).

231

The present work

The only situation indicated by our work as being one in which transference interpretations may become a danger to brief psychotherapy is when the therapist makes a persistent attempt to work through dependence in primitive 'two-person' terms with a patient who is deeply depressed. This happened in the second stage of therapy in the Hypertensive Housewife, and in the Car Lady (not considered in the present study) who was treated by the same therapist. The outcome in the case of the Car Lady was failure to terminate; while the Hypertensive Housewife became so depressed that she had to be admitted to hospital.

Apart from the special case mentioned above, the evidence thus suggests the opposite of our original fears: not only that transference interpretations do not intensify dependence, but even that the more successful cases tend to be those in which dependence does develop, though of course in moderation.

CHAPTER 12

The Exploration of a more 'Objective' Quantitative Approach to the Relation between Technique and Outcome

PRINCIPLES

Although the hypotheses presented in the preceding chapter may be felt to be quite convincing, and in a sense are based on published evidence, they depend entirely on the acceptance of very highly condensed summaries—themselves based on the therapists' own summaries—as an accurate reflection of what 'really' happened in these therapies. It must of course be remembered that I was able to draw not only on the clinical records, but also on the very vivid impression (for those cases not treated by myself) which can be given of the therapeutic process in a living discussion with the therapist, and on transcripts of the discussions taken down in shorthand at the time. Nevertheless, this double process of selection must be regarded as highly unsatisfactory.

It occured to me therefore that it might be worth while to explore the results given by some sort of 'content analysis' of the written case records, even though they themselves are the highly subjective productions of individual therapists. This would at least remove the second process of selection, and might partly answer the obvious criticism of the hypotheses reached in the preceding chapter, that they are produced by a single observer studying his own clinical judgements—which can obviously be used to lead in any direction that the observer chooses. If, after the second process of selection has been removed, something could be plausibly said about the factors at work in the first— i.e. about how the therapist selected the material that he recorded —then such a study might be brought much closer to what 'really' happened in therapy than the data which have been presented hitherto.

Since in Chapter 11 the main subject under study has been the attention paid by the therapist to interpretation of various aspects of transference, the obvious kind of study to begin with would be concerned with a purely quantitative measure of transference interpretation. In order to allow for the effects produced by the different lengths of these therapies and differences in the style and completeness of recording, the measure used would have to be a *proportion*—for instance, as a measure of 'transference orientation' we could use the ratio of the number of 'transference interpretations' to the total number of interpretations recorded. The kind of hypothesis which could be tested by such a study would be not of the form: 'the higher the proportion of a given kind of interpretation in the *therapy*, the more successful does the therapy tend to be,' but rather of the form: 'the higher the proportion of a given kind of interpretation in the *case record*, the more does the case record tend to be that of a successful therapy.'

There are many objections to such a study. The most obvious is that, since—for all we know—a single correct and well-timed interpretation may be all that is needed for a successful result, and therapists may persist with incorrect or inappropriate interpretations for hours, and since no account whatsoever would be taken of the response to the interpretation, any correlation between outcome and a purely quantitative measure of interpretation might be thought to be clinically meaningless. Would this not be yet another example of the 'ridiculous pseudo-rigor of those who count irrelevant entities simply to report that something has been counted' (Colby, 1960, p. 15)? I should like to ask the reader to adopt a different attitude: namely that it is not at all clear what the clinical significance of the study will be, but that it is worth suspending judgement until the results have been presented.

There are many other objections, however, which must be mentioned first. The case records vary widely in quality, and three of them are not complete. The effects of this will be considered in the appropriate place. Both the judgements of outcome and the judgements of the quantitative measures of interpretation have to be made by myself. I have partly met this by checking some of my own judgements against those made by an independent observer. Finally, the therapists were aware of some of the hypotheses to be tested, which may well have influenced the material that they have recorded. This also will be considered in the appropriate place. The one scientific advantage which the study can claim is that, since the idea for content analysis only came to me long after these therapies had been completed, the study is 'blind' in the sense that the therapists (including myself) were quite unaware at the time of recording of the approach that was going to be used.

An indication that the idea is not quite as absurd as it may sound may be obtained from the very interesting paper by Vosburg (op. cit. 1958) which has already been mentioned in connection both with fluctuations in motivation and with the inevitable development of transference (pp. 196–7 and 201). I was quite unaware of Vosburg's study until after much of my own had been completed. Vosburg carried out an analysis of the *style* of twenty-six case records ('hospital charts') of psychotherapy conducted by little-trained residents at the Western Psychiatric Institute of the University of Pittsburgh. These records were dictated from memory, and the record of one session averaged perhaps 'half a page of single-spaced typing in length'. He quickly realized, of course, that these notes obviously could not be regarded as 'objective' records of the content of the therapies, but that in some ways they were more valuable than objective records, because they were *dynamically* produced (by the therapists), and hence their style reflected highly relevant aspects of what was happening between therapist and patient. In consequence, it transpired, this style was correlated with outcome. 'On the basis of the enthusiasm, choice of words, suggestive phrases, and explicit remarks recorded in the hospital charts four styles of charts can be separated. This grouping was found to have a relation to the duration of treatment and to its outcome. . . . The hospital chart written in an *interactive style* is one which shows continuity of therapeutic remarks from hour to hour and records frequent interchanges between the doctor and patient. This group . . . includes the most successful results. . . . The hospital chart which sustains a language of remoteness and generalizations of the interview material may be characterized as a *remote style*. . . . There were no improvements recorded in this group.'

The important principle which Vosburg used—a principle always advocated by Balint and repeatedly emphasized in this book—is to regard all occurrences connected with a therapy—those initiated by the therapist as well as by the patient—as a result of a dynamic interaction between the two. A content analysis of the case records, regarded in this light, may thus well have a discoverable meaning.

The classification of styles which was used by Vosburg is not relevant to the case records in the present study, because with one possible exception all were written in a style which Vosburg would describe as 'interactive'. The exception is the Hypertensive Housewife, in whose record it is not easy to make out what was said by the therapist, and which therefore has to be omitted. The

235

studies that follow, therefore, were carried out (unless otherwise stated) on the remaining eighteen therapies.

For present purposes I propose to concentrate entirely on the content of the interventions made by the therapist, i.e. on interpretations. This requires operational definitions.

The idea for this study was originally suggested by the writings of Strupp, whose papers on content analysis have now been brought together in a book (Strupp, 1960). Since I had not read Strupp's work carefully, however, I worked out my own definitions, and arrived independently at several which are very similar to his. The formal statement of these definitions, and the principles on which the study has been carried out, will now be given. The result is somewhat more complicated than might have been expected originally.

Nearly all these case histories are written in a narrative style, of which the long quotations already given are fairly typical. A single (verbal) 'intervention' by the therapist is defined as a passage, however long and containing however many different elements, in which what the therapist said is reported, lying between two passages in which what the patient said is reported (this brief way of phrasing the definition is adapted from Strupp).

The technique used was almost entirely interpretative and interventions are therefore divided into only two classes:

1. *Interpretations*. An interpretation is defined as an intervention in which the therapist suggests or implies an emotional content in the patient over and above what the patient has already openly stated. Interpretations can be in the form of a question. An example of a 'borderline' interpretation—implying just a little more than the patient said—which is also in the form of a question, is shown below:

Patient: 'Seems so horrible to put a body into the earth to rot.'
Therapist: 'A feeling of desecration of the human body in some way?'

2. *Non-interpretative interventions*. In the present material these include exploratory questions, discussion of reality (such as times of appointments or length of treatment), answers to questions, and, very rarely, advice and reassurance.

Now an interpretation can be 'directed' towards some 'person', or can be 'undirected' (UD) which latter is taken to include those which are directed towards the self or towards some inanimate object. Three broad categories of person are considered:

236

1. Parent (P). Father or mother (in one case, stepmother).
2. Therapist (Th). This includes a previous therapist; and also 'treatment', 'clinic', or 'hospital' where obvious 'transference' feelings are involved.
3. 'Non-parent' (NP). This includes all people in the present or the past other than those in the two categories above.

It is necessary to digress here to discuss the clinical significance of the category 'non-parent'. It might be thought that this category should be restricted to, say, people of obvious emotional significance to the patient—e.g. marriage partner, boy or girl friend, sibling or child. In fact this would deny the intense emotional significance of apparently much less close relationships —such as that between the Lighterman and his employers (representing his mother who made him work in the house when he was a boy), or between the Articled Accountant and his boss (representing the authoritarian father—a phantasy figure), or even between the Pilot's Wife and men in general. For this reason I have found it almost impossible to draw lines of demarcation which are anything but arbitrary, and I include in the category NP all people other than parents and therapists, including the patient's unborn baby, and even such broad categories as 'men', 'school', or 'employers'. Little emphasis will therefore be laid on this category, but it plays an important part as a rough 'control'.

So far everything is straightforward, but a complication arises in a passage of the following kind:

Surgeon's Daughter (*session 1*): 'At this point . . . she said "He [her father] seemed to have no understanding of what I wanted." At this point I remarked on how like this was to the present predicament [i.e. that the therapist had no understanding of what she wanted].'

On the face of it, although this interpretation clearly introduces something new in the patient's relation with the therapist, it introduces nothing which the patient has not already openly stated in the relation with the patient's father. Yet clearer thinking (which it took me several days to reach) shows that something new is in fact introduced in the relation with the father, namely the *link* between feelings about the father and feelings about the therapist. This kind of interpretation is therefore considered to be directed both towards parent and towards therapist, and is scored PTh.

It will be clear that (as Strupp also emphasizes) every interpre-

237

tation has to be considered in the context of the material on which it is based, which makes the study of interpretations in isolation less one-sided than it may appear to be at first sight.

SCORING BY TWO INDEPENDENT JUDGES

The first essential is to check that these judgements are reproducible by more than one observer. Unfortunately, the heavy commitments of the other members of the team have made it impossible to check this as thoroughly as I would have wished, but one member—Mr. Eric Rayner, whose help I once more acknowledge with grateful thanks—undertook to learn the method of scoring and to carry it out independently on a total of five therapies. These therapies were deliberately chosen to represent four different therapists. Mr. Rayner's scoring took place long after I had completed my own for all these therapies. In order to keep the scoring simple, I asked him to consider only the following: (i) whether the intervention was or was not an interpretation, and (ii) whether it was directed towards parent, therapist, or 'other' (0). The category 0 thus contains my categories of NP (non-parent) and UD (undirected).

A comparison of his scorings with mine, in the order in which he carried them out and including the first which he tried, is shown in *Table 16*.

The two scorings of each therapy were compared and differences discussed after each had been carried out by Mr. Rayner. In the first two therapies which he scored there were several disagreements due entirely to Mr. Rayner's inexperience with the criteria used. (These largely account for the large difference in Th per cent between the two judges on the Surgeon's Daughter.) The scoring of each of us also exposed some slips in the other's work, and some judgements of our own with which on reconsideration we would have disagreed. *None of these errors has been corrected.* They are regarded as part of the experimental error inherent in any measurement.

It will be seen that (apart from the single large discrepancy mentioned above) the difference between the two judges on any proportion of P or Th never reaches 6 per cent. It must be emphasized that this is partly due to cancellation of differences; but for the purpose of the present study the agreement is regarded as satisfactory.

The proportion of judgements which are in agreement is in fact considerably smaller than that obtained by Strupp in his work. No doubt, if we had continued to confer carefully over the

TABLE 16 COMPARISON OF THE SCORING OF TWO INDEPENDENT JUDGES

Therapy	Therapist	Total number of interpretations Malan Rayner		Total number of judgements the same	Proportion¹ of judgements the same	Total involving P Malan Rayner		Proportion² involving P Malan Rayner		Total involving Th Malan Rayner		Proportion² involving Th Malan Rayner	
Surgeon's Daughter	C	38	40	29	71%	4	2	10%	5%	20	16	52%	40%
Unsuccessful Accountant	F	36	41	30	68%	0	0	0%	0%	25	28	69%	68%
Biologist	B	93	97	78	78%	27	26	29%	27%	17	23	18%	23%
Lighterman	F	78	79	70	86%	37	38	47%	48%	23	25	29%	32%
Student's Wife	G	52	47	41	76%	22	18	42%	38%	4	6	8%	13%

¹ The 'total' number of judgements' here is taken to be the total number of interventions scored by one or other of the two judges as an interpretation. Interventions judged by neither as an interpretation are not considered. This proportion is thus somewhat on the conservative side.

² Since some interpretations are judged as PTh the proportions involving P, Th, and O may add up to more than 100 per cent.

criteria used, we could ourselves have obtained a higher agreement. I would not, however, regard this as necessarily an advantage—since the criteria themselves are obviously a matter of opinion also. I would say that in fact this degree of agreement almost exactly reflects the accuracy of this type of measurement.

RESULTS OF THE COUNT OF INTERPRETATIONS

Some results of my own count of interpretations are shown in *Tables 17* and *18.*

TABLE 17 SOME RESULTS OF THE COUNT
OF INTERPRETATIONS

Patient	Total no. of sessions with Workshop member	Total no. of sessions recorded (if different from previous column)	Total no. of inter- pretations recorded	Average no. of inter- pretations per recorded session
Biologist	10		93	9·3
Lighterman	17 (incl. 1 session by emer- gency doctor in therapist's absence)		78	4·6
Neurasthenic's Husband	14	4 fully (first 2 and last 2. Rest summarized, but fairly fully.)	52	3·7
Falling Social Worker	40	14 fully (first 9, then irregularly. Rest briefly summarized and not included in this study.)	63	4·5
Railway Solicitor	30	11 (first 11. Rest not recorded.)	58	5·3
Girl with the Dreams	18 (not incl. independent assessment interview)		61	3·4

240

Table 17—*continued*

Patient	Total no. of sessions with Workshop member	Total no. of sessions recorded (if different from previous column)	Total no. of inter- pretations recorded	Average no. of inter- pretations per recorded session
Civil Servant	12 (not incl. independent assessment interview)		58	4·8
Surgeon's Daughter	18		38	2·1
Unsuccessful Accountant	7		36	5·1
Draper's Assistant	10		21	2·1
Storm Lady	19 (up to natural break in treatment)		285	15·0
Tom	4		17	4·2
Pilot's Wife	19		104	5·5
Student Thief	11		56	5·1
Paranoid Engineer	13 (up to point at which long- term therapy was agreed on)		44	3·4
Violet's Mother	15		64	4·3
Articled Accountant	27		213	7·9
Student's Wife	9	(Sessions 3 and 4 briefly summarized.)	52	5·8

TABLE 18 NO. OF INTERPRETATIONS PER RECORDED SESSION
ARRANGED ACCORDING TO THERAPIST AND OUTCOME

Therapist	Patient	Outcome	No. of interpretations per recorded session
A	Girl with the Dreams	2	3·4
	Civil Servant	1	4·8
	Draper's Assistant	0	2·1
B	Biologist	3	9·3
	Storm Lady	0	15·0
	Tom	0	4·2
C	Surgeon's Daughter	1	2·1
E	Neurasthenic's Husband	3	3·7
F	Lighterman	3	4·6
	Unsuccessful Accountant	1	5·1
	Pilot's Wife	0	5·5
	Student Thief	0	5·1
	Paranoid Engineer	0	3·4
	Violet's Mother	0	4·3
	Articled Accountant	0	7·9
G	Falling Social Worker	3	4·5
	Railway Solicitor	3	5·3
	Student's Wife	0	5·8

A more 'objective' quantitative approach

These two tables give the following results which are important in the interpretation of the later evidence:

1. A study of the relation between the *total number of interpretations recorded* and outcome shows a value of τ_b very slightly on the positive side of zero. This, however, is largely due to the presence of three unsuccessful therapies which were both long and very fully recorded (the Storm Lady, the Pilot's Wife, and the Articled Accountant). If these three therapies are excluded, the rest give a positive correlation which is 'significant' at the 5 per cent level. This is important, because it emphasizes once more the necessity for using ratios rather than absolute numbers in studies of the relation between outcome and any quantitative measure of different kinds of interpretation.

2. A study of the relation between the *average number of interpretations per recorded session* and outcome shows no trend whatsoever, the value of τ_b being very slightly negative. Nor is there any trend discernible for this variable between the more and the less successful cases treated by any individual therapist. This is a somewhat surprising result, because there is no question that therapists record more fully in a given therapy when a session occurs which is marked by intense communication. This is possible evidence that the overall intensity of communication, or the therapist's interest, by itself, is not correlated with successful outcome.

It is now necessary to consider the effect on the figures of the fact that three therapies (the Neurasthenic's Husband, the Falling Social Worker, and the Railway Solicitor) were incompletely recorded. I shall be concerned here with the broad categories of 'person' (mainly parent or therapist) towards whom the feelings in the interpretation were directed. Now it is a fortunate fact that in all three of these therapies the transference and the relation to parents were both interpreted from the very beginning, and continued to be so throughout therapy. In the Falling Social Worker and the Railway Solicitor there was a decrease in transference interpretation in the middle period of therapy, followed by an increase as termination approached (personal communication from the therapist). It is possible, therefore, that the figures obtained from the first third of therapy alone exaggerate the proportion of Th interpretations in the whole of therapy, but I doubt if this exaggeration is great. In the Neurasthenic's Husband, the therapist wrote on the termination form that 'the transference was intense from the first' and 'transference interpretations . . .

TABLE 19 PERCENTAGE ORIENTATION OF INTERPRETATIONS

Patient	Total no. of interpretations	Total UD	Total NP[1] oriented	Total P	Total Th	% UD	% NP	% P	% Th	Condensed percentages			
										UD	NP	P	Th
Biologist	93	24	39	28	17	26	42	30	18	30	40	30	20
Lighterman	78	15	32	37	23	19	41	47	29	20	40	50	30
Neurasthenic's Husband	52	1	39	17	31	2	75	33	60	0	70	30	60
Falling Social Worker	63	9	24	30	28	14	38	48	44	15	40	50	40
Railway Solicitor	58	12	10	20	35	21	17	34	60	20	15	30	60
Girl with the Dreams	61	20	21	18	14	33	34	29	23	30	30	30	20
Civil Servant	58	15	14	22	17	26	24	38	29	30	20	40	30
Surgeon's Daughter	38	5	23	4	20	13	60	10	53	15	60	10	50
Unsuccessful Accountant	36	5	21	0	25	14	58	0	69	15	60	0	70

Draper's Assistant	21	7	12	6	33	33	57	29	14	30	60	30	_15_
Storm Lady	285	177	42	14	39	62	15	14	14	60	_15_	_15_	_15_
Tom	17	5	2	11	1	29	12	65	6	30	_10_	60	_5_
Pilot's Wife	104	22	43	14	47	21	41	13	46	20	40	_15_	50
Student Thief	56	7	33	14	17	12	59	25	30	10	60	20	30
Paranoid Engineer	44	15	10	10	15	34	23	23	34	30	20	20	30
Violet's Mother	64	7	45	1	20	11	70	2	31	10	70	_0_	30
Articled Accountant	213	33	117	91	63	15	55	43	30	15	50	40	30
Student's Wife	52	9	31	22	4	17	60	42	8	15	60	40	_10_
Correlation with outcome $\begin{cases} \tau_b \\ p \end{cases}$										-0.07	-0.03	$+0.20$	$+0.36$ 0·069

¹ It should be noted that owing to the heterogeneous nature of NP the figures can only be approximate. They were also not checked by an independent observer.

were made in *every session*'. The proportion may be somewhat exaggerated by the last two intense transference sessions, but again not greatly. The therapy in the Falling Social Worker and the Railway Solicitor was also predominantly therapist-parent oriented, and in the Neurasthenic's Husband predominantly therapist-parent-non-parent oriented, throughout—so that again the general proportion of the three categories of interpretation would have been maintained. Since all these figures can never be anything but a rough guide, and since all results suggested by the figures are checked against clinical judgement, I do not believe that the errors introduced are in any way serious.

After this long preliminary, the reader is referred to the figures (*Table 19*).

It is necessary to note that since the unit under consideration is the 'interpretation' rather than (so to speak) the 'reference' to a given category of person, a single interpretation may be directed towards two or even all three of the categories of person considered, and therefore the figures for 'percentage orientation' of the three categories are not logically independent and may add up to more than 100—and indeed there is nothing, theoretically, to prevent them from adding up to 300.

COMPARISON OF THE TH RATIO WITH CLINICALLY
JUDGED TRANSFERENCE ORIENTATION

Before the figures are further considered, the 'Th ratio' or 'transference ratio' will be compared (*Table 20*) with the clinically judged four-point scale for 'transference orientation' which has already been considered. It must be remembered that the latter scale was reached long before the idea of counting interpretations had even occurred to me.

Inspection shows that, apart from the large discrepancy introduced by the Draper's Assistant (which has already been explained, see *Table 11*), agreement is fairly good. A correlation of the two scales gives $\tau_b = +0.60$ (including the Draper's Assistant but omitting the Hypertensive Housewife) for which $p = 0.003$. Of course, since there was a quantitative element in the 'transference orientation' judged clinically, it is not surprising that the correlation should be fairly high.

A comparison of the correlations with outcome given by the two methods is shown on page 248 below (the Hypertensive Housewife is omitted throughout).

TABLE 20 COMPARISON OF CLINICALLY JUDGED 'TRANSFERENCE ORIENTATION' WITH 'TH RATIO'

Patients in descending order of condensed Th ratio	Condensed Th ratio	Clinically judged transference orientation
Unsuccessful Accountant	70	3
Neurasthenic's Husband	60	3
Railway Solicitor	60	3
Surgeon's Daughter	50	2
Pilot's Wife	50	3
Falling Social Worker	40	3
Lighterman	30	2
Civil Servant	30	3
Student Thief	30	1
Paranoid Engineer	30	3
Violet's Mother	30	1
Articled Accountant	30	2
Biologist	20	1
Girl with the Dreams	20	2
Draper's Assistant	15	3?
Storm Lady	15	1
Student's Wife	10	0
Tom	5	0

The present work

	Clinically judged (four-point) 'transference orientation'	'Transference ratio'
(1) omitting the Draper's Assistant (17 patients)	$\tau_b = +0.37$ $p = 0.09$	$\tau_b = +0.32$ $p = 0.12$
(2) including the Draper's Assistant (18 patients)	$\tau_b = +0.30$ $p = 0.16$	$\tau_b = +0.36$ $p = 0.07$

The results given by the two methods are therefore not dissimilar, though the doubtful clinical judgement in the Draper's Assistant introduces a considerable discrepancy.

CORRELATION BETWEEN OUTCOME AND NP AND P RATIOS:
THE HYPOTHESIS OF THE THERAPIST-PARENT LINK

If the reader will now refer to the last three columns of *Table 19* once more, he will note:

1. that all proportions of NP, P, and Th which lie below 20 per cent (really below 17·5 per cent, since the figures in this range are given to the nearest 5 per cent) have been printed in italic type and underlined;
2. that there is a much higher proportion of figures in italic type in the less successful than in the more successful cases; and
3. that there is a suggestion that a low proportion of P (and not only of Th) is associated with a less favourable outcome; whereas
4. there is no evidence that such a relation applies to NP.

This suggests the possibility of the following clinical observation:

1. that, in this population, there was a tendency for those therapies that were both therapist- and parent-oriented to be the more successful; and
2. that therefore, possibly, those therapies tended to be more successful in which the link was made between the relation to the therapist and that to a parent, whereas the same does not apply to the link between therapist and non-parent.

Preliminary evidence tending to confirm this second hypothetical observation may be presented as follows:

1. In four of the five cases that score 3 for outcome (all except the Biologist), a major focus was the link between therapist and parents (it is worth noting how the 'hard core'—the Lighterman, the Neurasthenic's Husband, and the Falling Social Worker—appears once again):

Lighterman: (a) The link between therapist and father in session 3 (fear of being criticized for being a nuisance to his mother);
(b) The link between therapist and mother in sessions 11 and 14 (criticism of therapist and mother for not looking after him properly).

Neurasthenic's Husband: The two main foci of therapy were:
(a) Denigration of therapist and father; and
(b) Longing for therapist and father.

Falling Social Worker: Two of the main foci of therapy were:
(a) Sexual feelings for present therapist, previous therapist, and father; and
(b) Anger at therapist's and mother's indifference.

Railway Solicitor: The main focus in the first third of therapy was anxiety-laden rivalry with present therapist, previous therapist, and father.

2. In contrast, the therapies in which a main focus was the link between therapist and *non-parent*, and in which interpretations about the link between therapist and parent either were not made, or were little emphasized, or produced little response, were much less successful:

Score 1 for outcome (*valuable false solution*)

Unsuccessful Accountant: Here there were clear indications in session 2 that the patient's relation with his father was an important factor in his difficulties, and the possibility of using this in interpretations was envisaged in the original plan. In fact, the main focus was the link between tension in the sessions and tension before interviewing boards (non-parent), and the relation with the father was mentioned in no recorded interpretation.

Score 0 for outcome

Draper's Assistant: Although it is very difficult to know exactly what happened here, it was always my judgement (at the time that therapy was thought to have been successful) that the interpretation in session 6 (that the patient had to control therapist and husband) had been the main therapeutic factor. In any case, this link was made in this session, and no link to parent was recorded at any time.

Pilot's Wife: Here, again, there were clear indications that the patient's highly ambivalent relation to men was derived from that with her father. The link between therapist and *husband* was repeatedly made, and it was the therapist's aim to carry this further and make the link to the father. Although he did so in three interpretations, the patient's response was denial on all three occasions.

Violet's Mother: Here the original focus was interpretation of the patient's part in the family tension. When termination became an issue the disappointment in the therapist was repeatedly linked to disappointment with the husband, but the link to parents was never once mentioned in recorded interpretations.

This preliminary evidence leads at once to a formal statement of *the hypothesis of the therapist-parent link*:

That, in general, in these therapies, a necessary condition for success is that interpretation of the link between the transference and the patient's relation to one or both parents should become a major issue.

Now the link between the transference and the patient's *childhood* is universally recognized by psycho-analysts to be an essential factor in technique. Glover (1955, pp. 132, 133) writes:

'. . . we are never finished with a transference interpretation until it is finally brought home to roost. To establish the existence of a transference-phantasy is only half our work; it must be detached once more and brought into direct association with infantile life.'

'Transference experience and interpretation provide an affective experience (an affect-bridge) to link the past with the present.'

And Alexander, in *Psychoanalysis and Psychotherapy* (1957, p. 68) says:

'Interpretations which connect the *actual life situation* with *past experiences* and with the *transference situation*—since the latter is always the axis around which such connections can best be made—are called *total interpretations*. The more that interpretations approximate this principle of totality the more they fulfill their double purpose: they accelerate the assimilation of new material by the ego and mobilize further unconscious material.'

The link between transference and the patient's feelings about a parent does not necessarily bring in the patient's childhood, but it will necessarily have overtones connected with childhood. The confirmation of this hypothesis would therefore establish for brief psychotherapy a principle which is related to one long accepted for psycho-analysis.

Before the evidence is presented, some preliminary remarks must be made about linking interpretations in general. An interpretation linking the patient's feelings about one category of person (Th) to another category (P) can be of two main kinds which do not hold the same clinical significance:

1. The patient has already said something openly about the parent, and the therapist now links this with himself:

Surgeon's Daughter (*session 1*): [Patient says that] 'In fact she [patient] has not seen him [her father] . . . since having a shattering row with him at the time when she needed some counselling. . . .'

Therapist's report continues: 'I suggested to her that she felt she was in need of counselling again and was afraid that she might be faced with a shattering row.'

2. The therapist brings out by interpretation something in the relation to him, and then links this with the relation with the parent:

Neurasthenic's Husband (*session 13*): '. . . I pointed out to him his wish to become independent of psychiatric aid, to owe nothing at all to anybody, not to need me, to have no father, no psychotherapist, nobody, and thus to deny our potency.'

(The third kind of interpretation, in which the patient says something openly about the therapist, who then relates this to the parent, will not be distinguished from the second.)

251

TABLE 21 CLINICAL EVIDENCE ON THE THERAPIST-PARENT LINK

Patient	Score for outcome	Clinical evidence
A. THERAPIES IN WHICH THE THERAPIST-PARENT LINK WAS UNQUESTIONABLY A MAJOR ISSUE		
Lighterman	3	The link therapist-father (fear of being criticized for being a nuisance to his mother) produced a dramatic response in session 3. At two later important moments in therapy (sessions 11 and 14), when the patient came up in a state of anxiety which was resolved by interpretations of his anger with the therapist, the link was made with the patient's anger with his mother. This anger with his mother and the guilt about it were the main focus of the whole therapy.
Neurasthenic's Husband	3	The main focus of therapy was denigration of, and identification with, the patient's father. The link between the therapist and father was repeatedly made throughout the whole of therapy, and particularly in the moments of dramatic response to interpretation in sessions 13 and 14.
Falling Social Worker	3	Two of the main foci of therapy were: (i) The sexualized transference to the present and previous therapists, which was repeatedly linked to the patient's father. The link was made in session 10, when the patient expressed this transference by a vivid sexual phantasy about the therapist. (ii) Anger at the therapist's indifference during the patient's illness, which led at once to the exploration of similar feelings in relation to the patient's mother (session 30). Anger and grief at termination were also linked with the mother.
Railway Solicitor	3	Here the guilt- and anxiety-laden rivalry with men was repeatedly interpreted in relation to the therapist and linked to the father in the first 11 sessions. The patient clearly worked with this problem, though he did not respond dramatically to interpretation at any time.

Civil Servant	1	The main focus of the first 8 sessions was the fear of disagreeing with the therapist as father. This disagreement was brought into the open in session 7.
Student Thief	0	The clearest response to interpretation was in session 9, when the therapist resolved a tense situation by bringing out the patient's resentment at his taking for granted that she could come when it suited him. This was immediately related to problems of giving and taking in her relation with her mother and fiancé, which had been the focus of the whole therapy.
Articled Accountant	0	The wish for a permanent relation with the therapist to replace the lost relation with the patient's father was interpreted several times in sessions 4–7. When termination was threatened, almost the whole of therapy was directed towards interpreting anger about the loss of the therapist. This was repeatedly related to anger about loss of both parents in sessions 17–25.

B. INTERMEDIATE CASES: THOSE IN WHICH THE LINK WAS MADE ON ONE OR VERY FEW OCCASIONS, BUT THERE IS EVIDENCE THAT THIS HAD SOME IMPACT ON THE PATIENT

| Girl with the Dreams | 2 | Although the conflicting feelings about the therapist representing the patient's mother were the main issue in the second half of therapy, it seems both from the case notes and from the transcripts of the discussions that the link between therapist and mother was not often specifically made. There are in fact two places in the case notes where this was done, and one in which the link was made to the father. In the last session the link to the mother was based on a transparent dream, and the patient clearly understood and worked with the interpretation. The dream was of a woman with the same Christian name as the therapist, who had wept when she saw the patient (who was—in reality—pregnant) . . . 'and somebody had said, "Well . . . she wants to have a baby and she sees you with a swollen tummy".' The therapist's account continues: 'She went on from there after I had made the obvious interpretation, talking about my (her mother's)[1] jealousy.' |

[1] In brackets in the notes exactly as shown here.

Table 21—continued

Patient	Score for outcome	Clinical evidence
Surgeon's Daughter	1	Apart from two interpretations in session 1, in which the therapist linked what the patient had already said openly about her father to himself, there is only one interpretation (session 8) in which a clear link was made between therapist and father, but this was connected with the main focus and brought a clear response: 'I put it to her that she felt that her treatment would end soon and she would be put out, as by Dick and father, and that she felt bound hand and foot here, not being able to demand what she wanted. At this point she broke down and cried copiously....'

C. THERAPIES IN WHICH THE THERAPIST-PARENT LINK WAS MADE ON ONE OR VERY FEW OCCASIONS, AND THERE IS LITTLE EVIDENCE THAT THIS HAD MUCH IMPACT ON THE PATIENT

Patient	Score for outcome	Clinical evidence
Biologist	3	One interpretation in the last session: 'Also interpret his anxieties about leaving me in terms of going out into the world no longer with the support of a good strong father.' No response to this is recorded.
Pilot's Wife	0	There were three recorded interpretations making the therapist-parent link, to all of which the patient's response was denial.
Student's Wife	0	One interpretation making the link between therapist and mother is recorded, and the response was clearly doubtful: (Session 1) 'I tried to show her that she was asking me for all sorts of things which she really wanted to ask her mother for. . . .' This line of interpretation was completely abandoned in subsequent sessions.

| Paranoid Engineer | 0 | Here there was a single interpretation linking therapist and father by implication, but the patient's response was denial. |
| Storm Lady | 0 | In this very fully recorded therapy (285 interpretations) there is a single passage, the meaning of which is not entirely clear, in which the link was made between guilt about masturbation in relation to the parents and to the therapist. This was followed, shortly afterwards, by the most dramatic moment in the whole therapy, the interpretation about rape. I can only use clinical judgement and say that I do not believe this therapist-parent link had any significance in therapy. The link between *sexual* feelings for the therapist and the patient's father was not made at any time. |

D. THERAPIES IN WHICH THERE IS NO RECORD OF ANY INTERPRETATION OF THE THERAPIST-PARENT LINK, AND NO REASON TO SUPPOSE THAT SUCH AN INTERPRETATION WAS EVER MADE

Unsuccessful Accountant	1
Draper's Assistant	0
Tom	0
Violet's Mother	0

TABLE 22 SUMMARY OF EVIDENCE SHOWN IN TABLE 21
(IMPORTANCE OF THERAPIST-PARENT LINK—OUTCOME)

A	Score for outcome	B	Score for outcome	C	Score for outcome	D	Score for outcome
Lighterman	3	Girl with the Dreams	2	Biologist	3	Unsuccessful Accountant	1
Neurasthenic's Husband	3	Surgeon's Daughter	1	Storm Lady	0	Draper's Assistant	0
Falling Social Worker	3			Pilot's Wife	0	Tom	0
Railway Solicitor	3			Paranoid Engineer	0	Violet's Mother	0
Civil Servant	1			Student's Wife	0		
Student Thief	0						
Articled Accountant	0						

$$\tau_b = +0\cdot46 \quad p = 0\cdot03$$

A Therapies in which the therapist-parent link was unquestionably a major issue.
B Intermediate cases: those in which the link was made on only one or very few occasions, but there is evidence that this had some impact on the patient.
C Therapies in which the therapist-parent link was made on one or very few occasions, and there is little evidence that this had much impact on the patient.
D Therapies in which there is no record of any interpretation of the therapist-parent link, and no reason to suppose that such an interpretation was ever made.

TABLE 23 TRANSFERENCE ORIENTATION—OUTCOME ARRANGED AS IN TABLE 22

Score for transference orientation 3	Score for outcome	Score for transference orientation 2	Score for outcome	Score for transference orientation 1	Score for outcome	Score for transference orientation 0	Score for outcome
Neurasthenic's Husband	3	Lighterman	3	Biologist	3	Tom	0
Falling Social Worker	3	Girl with the Dreams	3	Storm Lady	2	Student's Wife	0
Railway Solicitor	3	Surgeon's Daughter	3	Student Thief	1		
Civil Servant	1	Articled Accountant	1	Violet's Mother	0		
Unsuccessful Accountant	1						
Pilot's Wife	0						
Paranoid Engineer	0						
(Draper's Assistant?)	0						

$\tau_b = +0.30$ $p = 0.16$

The second kind of interpretation would be expected to have a greater clinical significance than the first.

The clinical evidence for the hypothesis of the therapist-parent link is shown in *Table 21* and summarized in *Table 22*.

If it be thought arbitrary to make a distinction between a few recorded interpretations to which there was little response and no recorded interpretations at all, then categories *C* and *D* may be combined. In this case τ_b becomes $+0{\cdot}50$ and $p = 0{\cdot}02$.

Table 12, which shows the relation between transference orientation in general and outcome, may be arranged in the same form for comparison with *Table 22* (the Hypertensive Housewife is omitted). See *Table 23*.

The correlation with outcome shown by the therapist-parent link is thus very much greater than that shown by transference orientation alone; but clinical considerations reduce this difference considerably. The original judgement of high transference orientation in the Draper's Assistant may well be wrong, and therefore it is probably best if this patient is omitted. The correlations are then as below:

Comparison of clinically judged 'transference orientation' and 'importance of therapist-parent link' on seventeen cases (omitting the Hypertensive Housewife and the Draper's Assistant)

Correlations with outcome

	Clinically judged (4-point) 'transference orientation'	Clinically judged (4-point) 'importance of therapist-parent link'
τ_b	$+0{\cdot}37$	$+0{\cdot}43$
p	$0{\cdot}09$	$0{\cdot}05$

Since it has already been shown how sensitive these figures are to small changes in the scoring, this difference is far too small to point to any definite conclusion; and since there is no clinical way of separating the importance of the 'pure' transference interpretations from that of interpretations making the therapist-parent link, the study so far must be regarded as inconclusive. (Of course, if the Draper's Assistant is included, the difference is made far greater, and the result more strongly favours the therapist-parent link.)

Nevertheless, a different way of looking at the data does lead in the same direction more definitely. A *purely qualitative* consideration of transference interpretation—i.e. of whether or not there was at any point in therapy a clear response to such an interpretation—gives a distribution as below on the 2×2 contingency table (omitting the Hypertensive Housewife and the Draper's Assistant once more):

	Transference interpretation	
Outcome	*Response*	*No response*
3, 2, or 1	9	0
0	6	2

Without the additional evidence from the two patients omitted, this distribution can hardly be described as even suggestive. If the same considerations are now applied to the interpretation of the therapist-parent link, however, the distribution is as below:

	Therapist-parent link	
Outcome	*Response*	*No response*
3, 2, or 1	7	2
0	2	6

Although this distribution looks quite impressive, it is in fact only 'significant' at the 10 per cent level by the Fisher test (two-tailed). Nevertheless, it is far more suggestive than the distribution obtained by consideration of the response to transference interpretation alone.

Now of course the data presented above depend on a number of clinical judgements which are only a matter of opinion. I have therefore undertaken the corresponding quantitative study, but will not give it in detail because it has not been checked by an independent observer and because a presentation of the whole evidence would be too long in this context.

It is necessary to make an operational definition of an interpretation which specifically makes or clearly implies the therapist-parent link, and to calculate the proportion of interpretations making this link (the 'therapist-parent ratio'). If this is condensed to a four-point or three-point scale, it gives a correlation with outcome very similar to that given by the four-point and three-point scales judged clinically. Moreover, with a quantitative study it is possible to obtain a figure for the proportion of 'pure' transference interpretations (by subtracting the 'therapist-parent ratio' from the overall 'transference ratio'). It is therefore possible to compare the correlations with outcome of the 'pure' transference ratio and the therapist-parent ratio. The result, as I have scored it, is given below:

Correlation with outcome

'Pure' transference ratio	Th-P ratio (4-point)	Th-P ratio (3-point)
$\tau_b = +0.29$	$\tau_b = +0.46$	$\tau_b = +0.45$
$p = 0.15$	$p = 0.03$	$p = 0.04$

It is here that the category 'non-parent' comes into its own to provide additional evidence as a rough 'control'. If all that is being shown in the correlation of the therapist-parent ratio with outcome is simply the correlation with the overall transference ratio in another form, then the correlation with the therapist-non-parent ratio should be of the same order of magnitude. In fact, the therapist-non-parent ratio (admittedly much more roughly scored) gives a correlation with outcome close to zero.

I offer this as some further—not properly documented—evidence in favour of the therapist-parent hypothesis.

TRANSFERENCE AND FOLLOW-UP

It is a well recognized fact in psycho-analysis that after termination a patient is often left with an 'unresolved transference' which causes disturbance in any further contact with the analyst, and will usually be regarded as the main factor in any subsequent relapse. A study of the behaviour of the patient over follow-up, in relation to the degree to which the transference was interpreted during therapy, should therefore be of interest.

Now there are two highly undesirable situations which may occur after termination, and which lie at opposite extremes: one is that the patient is left feeling resentful, and refuses further contact with the therapist; the other is that the patient is left extremely dependent on the therapist, tries to get in touch with him and to ask for further sessions or a further course of treatment, and—at the extreme—termination becomes impossible. The optimum situation clearly lies between these two extremes, and may be described in the following way: the patient is left moderately and sincerely grateful, makes no attempt to ask for further sessions, but comes willingly for follow-up and may occasionally write in order to let the therapist know how he is getting on. Between the two extremes there are many intermediate situations and many forms of 'acting out' which are well illustrated by our own cases.

The variations in behaviour among these eighteen patients after termination or attempted termination are so interesting that I give the evidence here in full:

1. *Patients in whom the behaviour after termination was optimum*

The following patients showed no wish for further treatment and no trace of 'acting out', got in touch with the therapist if they had promised to do so, answered all letters, and came (when possible for practical reasons) to all appointments offered:

Falling Social Worker. This patient had returned to the west of England, where she worked, and had promised to get in touch with the therapist when she had a chance to come to London, three months after termination. She did so, and came to the appointment offered. At 1 year 7/12, in reply to a letter from the therapist, she gave the dates when she would be in London again, and came to the appointment offered. At 3 years, she gave a full and helpful reply to a letter of inquiry from the therapist.

Railway Solicitor. The final arrangement was that he would write to the therapist when he was next in London and would ask for an appointment. He did so and came to the appointment offered (2/12). At 5/12 he wrote spontaneously to the therapist when he passed his final examinations. At 7/12 he replied fully and helpfully to a letter of inquiry. The therapist replied that he would be happy to see the patient in the spring. The patient wrote (1 year 1/12) saying that he would be in London, but the therapist was on holiday. The therapist promised to get in touch with him, but did not do so. There were further helpful replies to letters of inquiry at 1 year 10/12, 3 years 4/12, and 3 years 8/12.

Surgeon's Daughter. She came to the appointment offered by the therapist (5/12). She wrote spontaneously at 10/12, opening the letter 'I am afraid I should have written to you a long time ago,

I don't really know what prevented me . . .' She then came to two appointments offered by an independent assessor (1 year, 2 years).

Unsuccessful Accountant. This patient spontaneously wrote a 'progress report' at 1/12; came for interview at 10/12; attended for a re-test at 1 year; and came for a further interview at 2 years.

Pilot's Wife. Here it was the therapist who 'acted out'—he had promised to get in touch with the patient at 3/12 and did not do so. Nevertheless the patient accepted and came to the first appointment offered (1 year). The therapist has not got in touch with the patient since.

Articled Accountant. He had promised to get in touch with the therapist 'in the autumn', about 6/12 after termination. At 3/12 his father died, he was extremely upset by this, and he felt tempted to ask for a further session. He did not do so, held out until the end of August or the beginning of September (date not recorded), and then rang the clinic. The therapist was away. He rang again after the therapist's return and came to the appointment offered (7/12). He came to a further appointment at 2 years 7/12.

2. *Patients in whom there was minimal to mild acting out*

Neurasthenic's Husband. This patient was offered his first follow-up interview at 5/12 by letter, *but delayed twelve days before replying.* He came to this appointment, however, and to one with an independent assessor; and subsequently to two further interviews (1 year 5/12, 3 years 3/12).

Civil Servant. An appointment had been made, during therapy, for 3/12 after termination, to which the patient came. At 1 year 1/12 he gave a useful reply to a letter from the therapist but wrote that he would *rather not come to see her.* He came to a further appointment offered at 1 year 9/12, another at 2 years 6/12, and an interview with an independent assessor at 2 years 11/12.

3. *Patients in whom there was moderate to severe acting out*

Biologist. This patient was written to at 5/12 and asked whether he would like another appointment. He carried this letter around in his pocket for weeks and *never answered it.* He was then written to at 7/12, and replied six days later. He came to an appointment at 8/12, delayed because of his holiday. He came to further follow-up interviews at 3 years and 5 years.

Lighterman. The patient had arranged to ring the therapist after returning from holiday at 2/12, and did so. At 7/12 he replied to a letter offering an appointment, but said he could not come because his wife had just had a baby. He promised to get in touch again as soon as he could come, *but did not do so.* At 1 year 1/12 he was offered another appointment but *did not reply*, and again at 1 year 2/12 (his wife destroyed the second letter because he had been so upset by the first). Finally, at 1 year 7/12 the patient came to an appointment offered. He promised to get in touch again when he had a week off, but *failed to do so.* At 4 years he replied to a letter offering an appointment, saying 'as I am now so much better I do not feel I want to visit your clinic. . . .'

Girl with the Dreams. Therapy was terminated just before she was due to have her baby. She replied to the therapist's first letter (1/12) asking about the baby, saying that she would probably be in London at 3/12 and would come to see the therapist then. She *did not do so*, and *failed to reply* to a letter at 4/12. The therapist wrote again at 5/12. The patient replied *after 2/12 delay*, and came to the appointment offered. This resulted in a further course of therapy.

Draper's Assistant. This patient was written to ten days after termination and offered appointments for a follow-up and re-test at 3/12. The letter ended 'perhaps you will let me know if this suits you'. She *did not reply*, and had to be written to again just before the appointment. She replied that *she felt there was no need.* The therapist wrote offering another appointment, to which the patient came. She was offered a further interview at 2 years, to which she came. This resulted in a further course of treatment.

4. Patients who refused to return altogether or at least for a long period

Tom. This patient, after breaking off treatment, *refused to come near the clinic again* because his father lived nearby. He was taken on for treatment at another hospital, spent a year in a mental hospital, and finally at 3 years 3/12 he was advised by his GP to consult the clinic again, and did so.

Student Thief. The therapist wrote to the patient at 2/52 asking her to attend for a re-test and independent assessment. She replied (twelve days delay) saying that she could not get away from work but would be glad to see the *therapist* any time after work. She was then offered further appointments, wrote and accepted them, but *failed to attend.* There was further correspondence, with the final result that the patient failed to answer. The clinic has *completely lost touch with her.*

5. Patients with whom there was failure to terminate

Storm Lady. Therapy was interrupted because the patient was due to have her baby, and the patient said that she 'expects she would like to come back and continue treatment as soon as she can after the baby is born'. She rang up the clinic at 2/12 asking for an appointment. This resulted in long-term therapy with the original therapist.

Paranoid Engineer. The original course of eight sessions came to an end when the therapist had to leave the clinic. Nevertheless, the patient was then seen irregularly. After initial improvement he relapsed, and the therapist finally agreed to see him once in three weeks indefinitely.

6. Patients referred for treatment elsewhere

Violet's Mother. There was relapse at threat of termination and the patient was referred to group treatment. The patient was compelled by circumstances to leave this group, and at 5/12 asked for an appointment with the original therapist who was 'the only person who had shared all this misery with her'.

Student's Wife. Therapy was terminated by the patient's departure for America. The patient has several times written to the therapist since to ask for his help in getting psychotherapy near where she lives.

7. Patients omitted from this study because they were omitted from the quantitative study of interpretations

Hypertensive Housewife (failure to terminate).
Clown (treated elsewhere).
Dog Lady (referred to group treatment).

The first five categories of behaviour after termination (or attempted termination) are shown in relation to transference ratio in *Table 24*.

The results shown in *Table 24* are the most striking in the whole of this study, and are perhaps the only results which would stand alone, unsupported by cumulative evidence from other sources. In summary, it can be said:

1. That of the six patients with the highest transference ratio, five showed optimum behaviour after termination and one the very mildest of acting out (delaying twelve days before answering a letter offering an appointment).

2. That the behaviour indicating either (a) excessive dependence on the therapist, or (b) a disturbance in the relationship resulting

TABLE 24 TRANSFERENCE RATIO IN RELATION TO TERMINATION AND FOLLOW-UP

Transference ratio	Failure to terminate	Optimum behaviour	Minimum to mild acting out	Moderate to severe acting out	Refusal of follow-up
70		Unsuccessful Accountant			
60		Railway Solicitor	Neurasthenic's Husband		
50		{ Surgeon's Daughter { Pilot's Wife			
40		Falling Social Worker			
30	Paranoid Engineer	Articled Accountant	Civil Servant	Lighterman	Student Thief
20				{ Girl with the Dreams { Biologist	
15	Storm Lady			Draper's Assistant	
5	OVER-DEPENDENCE	OPTIMUM RELATION	INCREASING DISTURBANCE		Tom

in severe acting out, occurred *entirely* in patients with a transference ratio of 30 per cent or less.

3. That a satisfactory relation with the therapist after termination, though clearly positively correlated with favourable outcome, is not as strongly correlated as might be expected—for instance, there are two patients scoring 0 for outcome who showed optimum behaviour, and two patients scoring 3 for outcome who showed moderate to severe acting out. It is clear, therefore, that this table indicates something more than merely the positive correlation between transference ratio and outcome already discussed.

In clinical terms, there is striking evidence: (i) that, on the one hand, thorough interpretation of the transference has a most beneficial effect on the patient's relation with the therapist after termination; and (ii) that, on the other hand, insufficient interpretation of the transference is likely to lead either to failure to terminate, or to disturbances in the relation after termination, with corresponding difficulty over follow-up.

Finally, there is an extraordinary contrast with the following passage from Stekel (op. cit. 1938) which I quote without comment simply because no obvious explanation of the discrepancy comes to mind:

'There will, then, be cases in which we shall hardly need to mention the transference, because it is not hindering but rather forwarding the analysis. It is in such analyses that we often get the best results. . . . The patient is grateful, keeps in touch when the analysis is over, writing or calling from time to time to ask for guidance upon some weighty decision. . . . But such cases are exceptional, and we usually find that the beginning of the transference proves the chief source of resistance.'

THE MEANING OF THE QUANTITATIVE STUDIES

So far in this chapter evidence has been provided in favour of certain hypotheses of the general form: 'A high quantitative emphasis on certain kinds of interpretation in the case records is associated with certain favourable aspects of outcome.' The question must be asked whether this really has any clinical significance at all.

The strong measure of agreement between the quantitative studies and the results of clinical judgement is only a partial argument; since, although for the clinical judgements I had the benefit of certain other sources of information (including, for my own cases, first-hand knowledge), I obviously also leaned heavily upon the case records themselves.

Now it is clearly impossible to be certain what relation the case records bear to the actual therapy. This much, however, can be said:

1. All the therapists were reasonably skilled, and the principle has always been used in this work that the therapist must on the whole be trusted.

2. Although the case records are highly selected, there are certain indications about factors in selection:

(a) The therapist tended to record more fully during sessions of intense communication (the evidence for this is very strong). Nevertheless, since there is no trend observable between outcome and number of interpretations per recorded session (even for an individual therapist, see *Tables 17* and *18*), it seems clear that the full recording of particular kinds of interpretation accompanying moments of intense communication cannot account by itself for any correlations observed.

(b) I do not believe that therapists were much influenced in their recording by the fact that certain hypotheses were under consideration—there is much evidence that therapists soon lost sight of hypotheses and plans in the heat of the therapeutic process.

(c) On the other hand, presumably therapists tended to lay greater emphasis on material and interpretations that fit in with psycho-analytic theory, or with well-established principles of psycho-analytic technique. This would apply to transference interpretations in general, and particularly to interpretations of the therapist-parent link, and would suggest that these interpretations have been 'concentrated' in these highly selected case records. In fact, there is direct evidence from the case records that this is true.

Yet this last argument does not weaken the clinical significance of the quantitative studies as much as might be supposed. If the therapist records a higher proportion of, say, therapist-parent interpretations because he believes in their efficacy, then he is unconsciously suggesting that therapy is going well, i.e. by implication making the prediction that outcome will be favourable; and in fact this prediction is borne out by subsequent follow-up—which is quite independent of his prediction. When he makes a similar unconscious prediction by recording more fully at moments of *any kind* of intense communication, on the other hand, his prediction is not confirmed.

To put this in another way, it may well be that there were two factors at work here: first, there was in fact a higher proportion of therapist-parent interpretations in the more successful therapies; and second, the therapist exaggerated this proportion by his method of recording. The two factors together then led to a much higher correlation with outcome than would have been given by either alone. Yet, again, this does not invalidate the clinical conclusion that these interpretations are important—for the therapies in which this double process occurred turned out, quite independently, to be the more successful. What this argument would suggest, on the other hand, is that the same clear correlation might not have been shown by tape-recordings.

The question may also be asked, what about the relative importance of *quantity* and *quality* of interpretations? The present results suggest that quantity is at least as important as quality; surely this is unlikely? Yet the answers to this question seem to me to be quite clear: (i) since the therapists are to be regarded as skilled, any interpretations that were frequently given (and not quickly abandoned) tended to be *appropriate*; (ii) an important interpretation almost always needs much preparative work before it can be given effectively; (iii) it is one of the principles of the 'focal' technique that therapist and patient together concentrate on a single theme in many different aspects throughout the whole of therapy; and finally (iv) surely what we are observing is one of the well-known lengthening factors, here kept within bounds, namely the necessity for *working through*. Direct evidence that important interpretations often have to be repeated can be seen most clearly in such cases as the Lighterman, the Neurasthenic's Husband, and the Pilot's Wife. Balint's idea (expressed in the early stages of the discussion on the Storm Lady) that you must 'take good aim and then fire' is essentially correct, but it seems that you need a number of 'ranging' shots first; and when you have found the range you must, so to speak, concentrate the whole battery upon the target.

THE STATUS OF THE EVIDENCE

At this stage there is a pressing need to survey all the evidence with a highly critical eye. Many arguments, some in favour of the evidence and some against it, will be presented and discussed.

First, the fact that this study was almost entirely retrospective can never be anything but a disadvantage. There are many warnings in the literature against regarding this kind of evidence as being more than provisional. One such warning was quoted on

p. 17, and it is worth while quoting another here. This is from Frank (op. cit. 1959):

'Perhaps the most important value of replication [i.e. cross-validation] is that it guards against *ex post facto* reasoning. There is no limit to the ingenuity of the human mind. It seems to be literally impossible to present a person with a set of data that are so random that he will not be able to read a relation into them. In psychotherapy if an experiment seems to demonstrate a certain relationship between therapeutic variables and changes in the patient, the experimenter can always make an hypothesis to explain it. This is a necessary and desirable first step to further research. A common error, however, is to offer the observed relationship as proof of the hypothesis. This circular reasoning can be escaped only by making an explicit prediction on the basis of the hypothesis and then seeing if the prediction is borne out with a fresh sample.'

This is a difficulty of which I am well aware. I have never forgotten how Ronald Knox, in a satire on the Baconians,[1] proved conclusively by means of anagrams that Tennyson's 'In Memoriam' had really been written by Queen Victoria; and I have long felt that there was a warning in this for all of us who work in psychotherapy.

Nevertheless, it must be remembered that many advances in science have been made by *ex post facto* reasoning; and whether or not it has been possible to repeat an observation, or to perform a new experiment based on prediction, has sometimes depended on quite accidental factors—for instance: in palaeontology, on whether a second specimen of a given fossil is ever discovered; or, in many branches of science, on whether most of the facts are already known before anyone thinks of a hypothesis to explain them.

This is not to say that cross-validation of the present results is not necessary; only that the evidence from *ex post facto* reasoning can be quite strong, if enough coincidences can be found in it. The present conclusions owe such force as they do possess not to a retrospective study of a single variable in a few cases, but essentially to convergence of evidence. The qualitative and quantitative studies, though not entirely independent, support each other; almost the whole of the evidence—as will be shown in the next chapter—can be reduced to a single fundamental principle; and finally, most of the individual hypotheses have been accepted for

[1] *Essays in Satire.*

269

years in a related method of psychotherapy, namely psycho-analysis.

In fact, we might well have derived our original hypotheses in a quite doctrinaire fashion from psycho-analysis, as one of our members, Goldblatt, did (if he will forgive me for saying so):

'If one believes, as I do, that one can only effect a permanent change in the patient by an analytic approach . . . then the question arises, if the principle of transference interpretation is correct, then it will be correct in treatment of the patient once a week, as well as in proper analysis.'

If we had consistently held this kind of view, our work could have been regarded as genuine cross-validation of fundamental psycho-analytic principles.

Against this, in turn, it must be said that the number of patients in this study is very small, lying towards the lower limit of the number for which statistical methods can be legitimately used for reaching any conclusions at all. I am well aware that the relapse of only two of the 'hard core' of successful cases would completely wreck almost all the correlations, though it would not have quite such a devastating effect on the hypotheses of the necessary condition. Moreover, further follow-up continues all the time, and the outcome of these therapies cannot be regarded as fixed. This is a second factor, in addition to the absence of cross-validation, that makes the evidence purely provisional.

One of the aims of the statistical approach has been to exclude entirely the disadvantage of 'clinical impression' about causality. It becomes very tempting to use the following type of argument: (i) this patient showed an improvement after a therapy in which a great deal of attention was paid to interpretation of the trans-ference; (ii) psycho-analytic experience makes me have more faith in transference interpretations than in any other kind of interpreta-tion; (iii) therefore transference interpretations were responsible for the improvement. Yet it must be admitted without shame that this kind of largely circular argument is present, reinforcing the purely statistical evidence presented.

Nevertheless, because an attempt has been made to exclude this kind of argument and to make the evidence less subjective, it is necessary to forestall another criticism; that the present study is really a piece of pseudo-objectivity far worse than pure 'clinical impressionism', because it gives the appearance of exactness and objectivity which is in reality quite illusory. In order to answer this, it is necessary to emphasize that the basic material of this study

270

consists almost entirely of clinical judgements. The aim has been not to pretend that these clinical judgements are objective or exactly quantitative, but simply to treat them—once they have been made—in as rigorous a way as possible, so that at least some fallacies can be excluded and the quality of the evidence can be partially assessed. It is one of the major purposes of the present study to suggest that this can in fact be done.

Again, what of the fact that the evidence presented consists almost entirely of a single worker's statistical study of correlations between his own clinical judgements? The disadvantages of the method are obvious, but there is an advantage also: that judgements made by someone who is prepared to give almost his whole time to them may possibly be made more self-consistent than the average taken from any number of judgements made superficially. This self-consistency may be attained only through profound thought, since each alteration in a judgement has repercussions among several others, and alterations in these may affect others, and so on. The result may be the necessity for a kind of free association spread over days or even weeks, accompanied —for me at any rate—by considerable mental distress.

Against this once more, it must be remembered that the criteria on which the judgements are based are themselves chosen subjectively, and may quite consciously be chosen so that the maximum correlation is obtained. Such a procedure is perfectly legitimate as long as the results are regarded as lying closer to hypotheses than to conclusions. Therefore the need to put the word 'significance' always in inverted commas is given further emphasis. It is worth re-stating that none of the correlations presented here is really significant in the statistical sense at all.

This leads to the question of cross-validation. In fact the material from at least forty further patients is available, and I have used some of it to check most of the hypotheses presented here by clinical impression, though certainly not in any rigorous way. Yet there is a complication. An extremely important characteristic of these early therapies is that they were not approached in any doctrinaire spirit, and thus were the genuine products of spontaneous interaction between therapist and patient. The failure of scientific discipline—such a disadvantage in the presentation of the evidence—was here an advantage, because the work was very little contaminated by the wish to prove or disprove a given hypothesis. Moreover, since no therapist was even aware, for instance, that the therapist-parent link, or work on termination, would prove to be important factors, no therapist made these kinds of interpretation unless they seemed to be indicated by the patient's material. Therapists who have become fully aware of these factors will be contaminated, and will show a tendency to make interpretations because they feel on theoretical grounds that therapy will not be successful unless they do, and not because the patient's material makes such interpretations necessary. This has almost certainly already happened with transference interpretations in general, and probably with interpretations about termination; though probably not to the same extent with the therapist-parent link, which has played a very small part in our discussions. The result will almost certainly be that the later population of therapies will be heavily selected in favour of high emphasis on transference interpretations, and that these interpretations will have been made whether the patient's material clearly indicated them or not. This will mean that the likelihood of obtaining high correlations (implying parallel variation) will be greatly reduced by the kind of 'exceptions' that do not contradict the hypothesis of the necessary condition. Whether there will be enough 'control' cases containing both clear communication (surely a necessary condition) and few transference interpretations remains to be seen.

CHAPTERS 11 AND 12: CONCLUSION

The importance of the evidence presented in Chapters 11 and 12 lies here: that whereas, in the Assessment and Therapy Forms and in the purely descriptive Chapter 10, it was shown simply that good therapeutic results could be obtained with a relatively fearless radical technique; in the two chapters under review it has been shown further that in these particular therapies, on the whole, the more radical the technique the better the results. Here, then, is some evidence to suggest that the two are in some way causally related.

CHAPTER 13

Recapitulation and Conclusion

The following is a formal summary of the work already presented:

GENERAL STATEMENT OF THE CHARACTERISTICS OF PATIENTS, THERAPISTS, AND TECHNIQUE

1. All patients were adults;[1] were thought to be highly suitable for psychotherapy; were willing and able to explore their feelings; gave the impression that they could work in interpretative therapy; and gave material at interview which was understandable in psycho-analytic terms and which enabled psycho-analysts to formulate some kind of limited therapeutic plan.

2. All therapists were psycho-analytically oriented, and were willing to employ a relatively 'active' technique which was entirely interpretative, was highly selective ('focal'), and in which emphasis was laid on 'objective' emotional interaction with the patient.

HYPOTHESES AND CONCLUSIONS ALREADY PRESENTED

1. Therapeutic results
Under the above conditions it is possible to obtain quite far-reaching improvements not merely in 'symptoms' but also in neurotic behaviour patterns, in patients with relatively extensive and long-standing neuroses.

2. Length of therapy
These results can be obtained in ten to forty sessions.

3. Selection criteria
(a) The hypothesis that it is the patients with 'mild' illnesses of recent onset who give the best results (Hypothesis A) is not supported.
(b) Our results suggest that—when the patients have already been

[1] One adolescent (Tom).

273

selected as described above—an important criterion indicating a good prognosis is concerned with a high motivation for insight therapy.

4. Characteristics of technique regarded as the result of interaction between patient and therapist
There is strong evidence:

(a) that thorough interpretation of the transference plays an important part in leading both to favourable outcome and to an optimum relationship with the therapist after termination;

(b) that important subdivisions of transference interpretation are (i) the negative transference, and (ii) the link between the transference and the relation to one or both parents; and

(c) that those therapies tend to be more successful in which transference interpretations become important early, and/or in which interpretations of the patient's grief and anger at termination are a major issue.

(d) Our work provides some slight evidence that therapists tend to be more successful early in their experience of this kind of therapy, when (presumably) their enthusiasm is highest.

A UNIFYING FACTOR

The essence of most of these hypotheses may now be repeated in the following words:

Prognosis seems to be most favourable when the following conditions apply: The patient has a high motivation; the therapist has a high enthusiasm; transference arises early and becomes a major feature of therapy; and grief and anger at termination are important issues.

Suddenly there crystallizes, from all the complexity of this long exposition of evidence, a single unifying factor of extraordinary simplicity:

That the prognosis is best when there is a willingness on the part of both patient and therapist to become *deeply involved*, and (in Balint's words) to bear the tension that inevitably ensues.

Obviously this must be qualified. Each must become involved in a special way: the patient must bring to the therapy his intense wish for help through insight, and to the relation with the therapist both his neurotic difficulties and some of his dependence —but dependence that is neither too intense nor too primitive; while the therapist must bring his human sympathy, his therapeutic enthusiasm, and his willingness to interact 'objectively', and he obviously must not become so involved that—for instance—he is resentful if therapy fails, and still less must *his* involvement be seriously complicated by unconscious reverberations from the past.

This willingness to become involved may well be an important 'non-specific' factor in psychotherapy, which our particular kind of therapy shares with many others. That such factors are needed to explain the apparently good therapeutic results obtained by such a large variety of techniques is becoming increasingly widely realized. In order to show that this particular factor may be important in types of therapy very different from our own, I only need to point to the work of Vosburg (op. cit. 1958) in which the presence of this factor in the *therapist* seemed to be a necessary condition to 'improvement' (though admittedly symptomatic improvement and without follow-up); and to the highly successful example of client-centred therapy reported by Rogers and Dymond ('Mrs. Oak'; op. cit. 1954) where it was unquestionably present in both therapist and patient. This is worth supporting by quotations:

From the transcript of the patient's first mention of the subject of termination:

'Yes I feel this dependency . . . it's comparable to the feeling you get when you're just finishing a very meaningful book, and have only a few pages left—a sort of wishing that you could prolong it. And there's regret, but still it's still with you, and you can still have it and touch it, and even give it away, and yet if need be go back to it.'

From the author's comments on the therapy:

'. . . for her, one of the deepest experiences in therapy . . . [was] the realization that the therapist *cared*, that it really mattered to him how therapy turned out for her. . . .'

The 'specific' factor in our kind of therapy seems to be a special variety of this involvement on the part of the patient, together with insight into its meaning; i.e. the transference experience accompanied by transference interpretation, and particularly the experience and interpretation of the negative transference and of the therapist-parent link.

SELECTION CRITERIA

Now it is tempting to draw, from these hypotheses, certain conclusions about *technique*: that the therapist should start making transference interpretations as soon as possible, should take every opportunity of making the therapist-parent link, and should always devote the last third or quarter of therapy to making interpretations about termination. Whereas I certainly agree that the therapist should be aware of these factors in technique as general principles, I suspect that there is implied here a mistaken judgement about the causal relations involved. It must be remembered that the hypotheses reached in the present work—whether by clinical judgement or statistically—are all based essentially on correlations. It is a characteristic of correlations that they give no information about causal relations—a positive correlation between two factors may occur if one causes the other, or vice versa, or if both are the results of a common cause. When this consideration is applied to the present data, it will become clear that the development of transference, and hence whether transference is interpretable, presumably depend more on factors in the patient than on factors in the therapist. There is plenty of evidence from our cases that the therapist is unable not only to prevent the development of transference, but also to make use of transference interpretations unless the patient is willing and ready to hear them. If the patient has no grief about leaving therapy (e.g. the Pilot's Wife), there is no point in interpreting it. In other words, the characteristics of successful therapy that have been described are at least as much concerned with selection criteria as with technique. This view, reached by myself after such laborious study of the data, has already been expressed intuitively in the Workshop:

> *Pines*: 'If we say this is the aim in short-term therapy—dealing as soon as possible with termination and breaking off dependency—we should take on patients who can quickly enter into relationship. We should say that this man was unsuitable because it took him a long time to reach this point.'

This suggests a new group of selection criteria:

1. the early development of transference, especially of a difficulty in the transference, and excluding, of course, certain kinds of transference;
2. the capacity to mourn (already postulated by Dicks in the preliminary discussions). It seems possible that this might be judged from projection tests.

Now it will be remembered that one of our original selection criteria was a 'history of real and good relationships', and two of the criteria used throughout this work by the psychologists in projection tests were the 'ability to tell stories about real people' and the 'ability to face emotional conflict'. Obviously all these criteria are closely related to the 'willingness to become involved and to bear the tension that ensues' which crystallizes from the present data. Yet none of these criteria proved of much value in predicting outcome. The question is, why?

The only tentative answers that I can give are, first, that the emphasis on 'real' may be mistaken. The relation with the therapist is of a unique kind, in which phantasies derived from the past are allowed free play, and it seems to be the willingness to express these in this relation which leads to a favourable outcome. Second, the judgements of the psychologists, like those of all of us, were always overshadowed by Hypothesis A, against which our data have provided such strong evidence. There is a great need for a re-examination of the material given by these patients in projection tests, to see if some factor connected with 'willingness to become involved' can be identified.

Because the patients in the present study represent such a highly selected population, there are certain selection criteria which may well be extremely important, but which have not been put to the test in our work at all. These consist of the characteristics which were shared by all the patients and which are listed on p. 273. If they are regarded, once more, as products of the interaction between patient and therapist, they may be re-stated in the following way:

1. The patient's willingness and ability to explore feelings;
2. The patient's ability to work within a therapeutic relationship based on interpretation;
3. The therapist's ability to feel that he understands the patient's problem in dynamic terms; and
4. The therapist's ability to formulate some kind of circumscribed therapeutic plan.

Here one can only say that undocumented experience and intuition both suggest that these four criteria may well come near to being necessary conditions to successful focal therapy.

A POSSIBLE FUTURE SELECTION PROCEDURE

The following procedure is now tentatively suggested as a way of making practical use of all the above considerations concerning selection criteria:

1. It is essential that partial interpretations should be made in the psychiatric interview. The purpose of this is (a) to make plain to

the patient that he will be offered interpretative therapy and very little else; (b) to gauge his ability to explore his feelings and his capacity for insight; and (c) to see what effect interpretations have upon his motivation.

2. For those patients who seem likely to be suitable, I would be inclined to recommend a second exploratory interview about a week later. The purpose of this is to give the patient a longer period during which his reactions to interpretative therapy can be studied.

3. The projection test is then given, about a week later than the second exploratory interview.

4. If (a) it is clear that the patient can be offered treatment of some kind, and (b) there is any doubt about his wish to come during this initial period, I would suggest that he should now be asked to think the situation over and write, saying whether he would like another appointment. If he does not write, or if there is a long delay before he does so, the prognosis is automatically regarded as bad.

5. The therapist and psychologist (and the group, if they are working in a group) confer, and see if they can understand the patient's problem and formulate a therapeutic plan.

6. Careful note is made of all fluctuations in motivation and all manifestations of transference during this period.

Indications of a good prognosis would then be:

(a) The material is understandable;
(b) A therapeutic plan can be formulated;
(c) There is some indication that the patient is beginning to work with interpretations;
(d) There are signs of developing transference—though, obviously, of a not too dependent or demanding kind; and
(e) Motivation either starts high or shows a rapid increase during this whole period.

The hypothetical working of this procedure may be illustrated by one of the cases in the present study, the Pilot's Wife (though the uncertain influence of the endocrine factor on this patient's prognosis introduces a complication). Her complaint was frigidity, her emotional problem an intense resentment against men, and she started to *interact* with her (male) interviewer before she ever saw him, demanding to be seen by a woman doctor. At interview and at test she presented the whole of her psychopathology; and

278

consequently there would have been no difficulty in formulating a therapeutic plan: to assign her to a male therapist, to interpret her resentment against men in the transference, and to relate this both to her frigidity and to a (presumed) highly ambivalent relation with her father. So far, all the signs were favourable. Nevertheless, her motivation was clearly ambivalent—on the one hand she said that she did not believe in psychiatry, and on the other she seemed prepared to go to some trouble to come. For this she should have been given the benefit of the doubt. When she was asked in the second interview to talk about whatever she liked, however, and she spent the whole session chatting about trivialities, the prognosis would become more doubtful. When she rang up five mintues before the third interview, wanting to put off treatment indefinitely because her husband had got into trouble, the prognosis would become very bad; and when, finally, six months later, she asked for treatment again, she either would have been referred elsewhere, or would have been accepted with the firm prediction that treatment would fail. In fact she was taken on and, in spite of a therapy of intense interaction throughout, she remained quite unchanged.

RELATION TO PREVIOUS WORK

It will be remembered from Chapter 3 that the literature on brief psychotherapy is marked by utter confusion, which can be summarized in the conflict between the conservative and the radical views. Our own views, starting well towards the conservative end of the spectrum, have ended by being probably more radical than those of any other authors except Thorne, somewhat more so even than those of Alexander and French. This has applied to every aspect of the field. According to our views: quite ill patients can be helped; apparently deep-seated neurotic behaviour patterns can be changed; transference interpretation is almost essential; the negative transference should not be feared but welcomed; it is quite safe—sometimes even necessary—to make 'deep' interpretations, to use dreams and phantasies, to make the link with childhood.

The question that immediately arises is: how cogent, and how universally applicable are the conclusions and hypotheses presented here? In my view it has been established:

1. that psycho-analytically based brief psychotherapy is possible;
2. that lasting improvements in neurotic behaviour patterns can be obtained in patients with moderately severe and long-standing illnesses;

3. that these results can be obtained with a technique which, apart from being active and 'focal', closely resembles that of psycho-analysis and deals fearlessly with most of the same issues; and

4. that such a technique carries few dangers if properly used.

The importance of these conclusions lies not in their being new, which to a large extent they are not, but in the fact that though they are clearly deducible from the literature they have never been widely accepted. The fault has lain on both sides: conservative preconceptions, fears, and prejudices have never been answered by radical evidence properly presented. There are several examples in the history of science of evidence which has been ignored, and has been rediscovered only when the world at large was ready to accept it.

Yet the other more tentative conclusions about selection criteria and the relation between technique and outcome—even if they later come to be more or less cross-validated—cannot necessarily be regarded as of universal application. Hypothesis A can still be statistically correct; far-reaching changes can still almost certainly be obtained without transference interpretation, e.g. in client-centred therapy. One of the main themes of the present study is that the whole course of therapy depends to a hitherto unrealized extent on subtle factors within both patient and therapist. In particular, a technique which is suitable for one kind of therapist is not necessarily suitable for another. Moreover, it is possible that technique itself may be less important, and certain non-specific factors such as unconditional acceptance of the patient more important, than has hitherto been realized (see Strupp, op. cit., pp. 319ff.). If this is so, it might even be that the only result of the correlation of technique with outcome presented here is to suggest that psycho-analysts—and indeed psycho-analysts with a special outlook within psycho-analysis itself—get the best results in brief psychotherapy when they use a technique which (always apart from passivity) most closely fits in with the basic principles in which they have been trained. No doubt the same, *mutatis mutandis*, would be shown by a similar study carried out by client-centred therapists. Nevertheless, for psycho-analysts alone this is an important conclusion, because it may help to free them from the constricting belief that a patient can only 'really' be helped by a full-scale analysis. Alexander and French challenged this view, and yet their work led to nothing but endless hostility and controversy—in my view purely because it was presented as a modification of psycho-analytic technique, instead of being presented as a technique of brief psychotherapy based on that of psycho-analysis. Balint deserves full credit for seeing that the whole question needed to be re-opened.

At the same time, the following word of warning is essential. One of our members (Mr. Rayner) said to me recently that he 'doubted if he could do focal therapy by himself'. It may well be that the system of working in a group, with a common purpose and enthusiasm, has had a very considerable influence on our results—comparable, indeed, with the possible effect on the results obtained by the early analysts of being members of a small and exclusive band of workers exploring a new field. Our own work has certainly suffered as enthusiasm has waned and as tensions have developed within the group. It is not necessarily true, therefore, that anyone can learn to apply the technique and expect to get the same results under entirely different conditions.

THE LENGTHENING FACTORS. THE PLACE OF THE PRESENT WORK IN THE HISTORY OF PSYCHO-ANALYSIS

There seems no question that almost all of the lengthening factors, which have played such an overwhelming part in the development of psycho-analytic technique, can in certain cases be counteracted or avoided. Thus *resistance, transference, dependence, negative transference, anger over termination*, and the *roots of neurosis in early childhood* can all simply be handled by direct interpretation; *passivity* and *therapeutic perfectionism* in the therapist, the *sense of timelessness, over-determination*, and the development of the *transference neurosis* can all be counteracted or avoided by frank discussion of the limits of therapy with the patient at the beginning, by the formulation of a plan and a limited therapeutic aim, and by the pursuit of this aim with the aid of the focal technique; and *working through*, though necessary, can be accomplished within the limits of a therapy which can still be described as 'brief'. Yet one factor has been left out and may well prove to be the most difficult to counteract of all. This, of course, is *waning enthusiasm*.

All that remains is to put this work into its historical perspective. It began with an attempt to turn back the clock and return to a primitive technique used by the early analysts and discredited for years. It has ended with the development of a technique derived from that used by analysts today. If only the problem of waning enthusiasm can be solved, such a development would seem far more likely to survive the test of time.

References

ALEXANDER, F. (1937). *Five-year report of the Chicago Institute for Psychoanalysis, 1932-37.*

ALEXANDER, F. (1944). Indications for psychoanalytic therapy. *Bull. N.Y. Acad. Med.* **20**, 319.

ALEXANDER, F. (1957). *Psychoanalysis and psychotherapy.* London: George Allen & Unwin.

ALEXANDER, F. and FRENCH, T. M. (1946). *Psychoanalytic therapy.* New York: Ronald Press Co.

BALINT, M. (1957). *The doctor, his patient, and the illness.* New York: International Universities Press; London: Pitman.

BARRON, F. (1953a). Some test correlates of response to psychotherapy. *J. cons. Psychol.* **17**, 235.

BARRON, F. (1953b). An ego-strength scale which predicts response to psychotherapy. *J. cons. Psychol.* **17**, 327.

BARRON, F. and LEARY, T. F. (1955). Changes in psychoneurotic patients with and without psychotherapy. *J. cons. Psychol.* **19**, 239.

BENNI, W. (1911). Ein Fall von Intestinalneurose. *Zbl. Psychoan.* **2**, 204.

BERLINER, B. (1941). Short psychoanalytic psychotherapy: its possibilities and its limitations. *Bull. Menninger Clin.* **5**, 204.

BINSWANGER, L. (1912). Analyse einer hysterischen Phobie. *Jb. psychoanal. psychopath. Forsch.* **3**, 228.

BREUER, J. and FREUD, S. (1895). Studies on Hysteria. *The complete psychological works of Sigmund Freud,* Vol. II. London: Hogarth (1955).

BRILL, A. A. (1910). Ein Fall von periodischer Depression psychogenen Ursprungs. *Zbl. Psychoan.* **1**, 158.

BRILL, N. Q. and BEEBE, G. W. (1955). *A follow-up study of war neuroses.* V. A. Medical Monograph.

CARMICHAEL, H. T. and MASSERMAN, J. H. (1939). Results of treatment in a psychiatric out-patient department: A follow-up study of 166 cases. *J. Amer. med. Ass.* **113**, 2292.

COLBY, K. M. (1960). *An introduction to psychoanalytic research.* New York: Basic Books.

CURRAN, D. (1937). The problem of assessing psychiatric treatment. *Lancet,* **ii**, 1005.

DATTNER, B. (1911). Eine psychoanalytische Studie an einem Stotterer. *Zbl. Psychoan.* **2**, 18.

DENCKER, S. J. (1958). A follow-up study of 128 closed head injuries in twins using co-twins as controls. *Acta psychiat. neurol. Scand.* **33,** Supplement 123.

DENKER, P. G. (1946). Results of the treatment of psycho-neurosis by the general practitioner. *N.Y. St. J. Med.* **46,** 2164.

DEUTSCH, F. (1949). *Applied psychoanalysis.* New York: Grune and Stratton.

EDER, D. M. (1911). A case of obsession and hysteria treated by the Freud psycho-analytic method. *Brit. med. J. ii,* 750.

ELLIS, A. (1957). Outcome of employing three techniques of psychotherapy. *J. clin. Psychol.* **13,** 344.

EYSENCK, H. J. (1952). The effects of psychotherapy, an evaluation. *J. cons. Psychol.* **16,** 319.

EYSENCK, H. J. (1960). *Handbook of abnormal psychology.* London: Pitman.

FENICHEL, O. (1930). *Ten years of the Berlin Psycho-analytic institute, 1920–1930.*

FERENCZI, S. (1920). The further development of an active therapy in psycho-analysis. In *Further contributions to the theory and technique of psycho-analysis.* Trans. J. Suttie. London: Hogarth (1950).

FERENCZI, S. (1925). Contra-indications to the 'active' psycho-analytic technique. In *Further contributions to the theory and technique of psycho-analysis.* Trans. J. Suttie. London: Hogarth (1950).

FERENCZI, S. and RANK, O. (1923). *Entwicklungsziele der Psycho-analyse; zur Wechselbeziehung von Theorie und Praxis.* Vienna, Leipzig, Zürich: Int. Psychoanal. Verlag.

FERENCZI, S. and RANK, O. (1925). *Development of psycho-analysis.* Trans. Newton, C. Nervous and Mental Disease Monographs, No. 40.

FINESINGER, J. E. (1948). Psychiatric interviewing. I. Some principles and procedures in insight therapy. *Amer. J. Psychiat.* **105,** 187.

FRANK, J. D. (1959). Problems of controls in psychotherapy as exemplified by the psychotherapy research project of the Phipps Clinic. In E. A. Rubinstein and M. B. Parloff (Eds.), *Research in psychotherapy.* American Psychological Association Publications.

FREUD, S. (1896). The aetiology of hysteria. In *The complete psychological works of Sigmund Freud,* Vol. III. London: Hogarth (1962).

References

FREUD, S. (1904). Freud's psycho-analytic procedure. In *The complete psychological works of Sigmund Freud*, Vol. VII. London: Hogarth (1953).

FREUD, S. (1905). Fragment of an analysis of a case of hysteria. In *The complete psychological works of Sigmund Freud*, Vol. VII. London: Hogarth (1953).

FREUD, S. (1909). Notes upon a case of obsessional neurosis. In *The complete psychological works of Sigmund Freud*, Vol. X. London: Hogarth (1955).

FREUD, S. (1912). The dynamics of transference. In *The complete psychological works of Sigmund Freud*, Vol. XII. London: Hogarth (1958).

FREUD, S. (1913). On beginning the treatment (Further recommendations on the technique of psycho-analysis, I). In *The complete psychological works of Sigmund Freud*, Vol. XII. London: Hogarth (1958).

FREUD, S. (1914). On the history of the psycho-analytic movement. In *The complete psychological works of Sigmund Freud*, Vol. XIV. London: Hogarth (1957).

FREUD, S. (1918). From the history of an infantile neurosis. In *The complete psychological works of Sigmund Freud*, Vol. XVII. London: Hogarth (1955).

FUERST, R. A. (1938). Problems of short time psychotherapy. *Amer. J. Orthopsychiat.* **8**, 260.

GLOVER, E. (1955). *The technique of psycho-analysis*. London: Baillière, Tindall & Cox.

GUTHEIL, E. (1933). Basic outline of the active psychoanalytic technique. *Psychoanal. Rev.* **20**, 53.

GUTHEIL, E. (1945). Psychoanalysis and brief psychotherapy. *J. Clin. Psychopath.* **6**, 207.

HUNTER, R. A. and MACALPINE, I. (1953). Follow-up study of a case treated in 1910 'by the Freud psycho-analytic method'. *Brit. J. med. Psychol.* **26**, 64.

JONES, E. (1953). *Sigmund Freud, Life and Work*, Vol. I. London: Hogarth.

JONES, E. (1955). *Sigmund Freud, Life and Work*, Vol. II. London: Hogarth.

KENDALL, M. G. (1955). *Rank correlation methods*. London: Charles Griffin.

KESSEL, L. and HYMAN, H. T. (1933). The value of psycho-analysis as a therapeutic procedure. *J. Amer. med. Ass.* **101**, 1612.

KNIGHT, R. P. (1937). Application of psychoanalytic concepts in psychotherapy. *Bull. Menninger Clin.* **1**, 99.

References

KNIGHT, R. P. (1941). Evaluation of the results of psychoanalytic therapy. *Amer. J. Psychiat.* **98**, 434.

LANDIS, C. (1938). Statistical evaluation of psychotherapeutic methods. In S. E. Hinsie (Ed.) *Concepts and problems of psychotherapy*, pp. 155-65. London: Heinemann.

LUFF, M. and GARROD, M. (1935). The after-results of psychotherapy in 500 adult cases. *Brit. med. J. ii*, 54.

MALAN, D. (1959). On assessing the results of psychotherapy. *Brit. J. med. Psychol.* **32**, 86.

MAUDSLEY HOSPITAL (1931). Medical Superintendent's Report. London: L.C.C. publication.

MILES, H., BARRABEE, E., and FINESINGER, J. (1951). Evaluation of psychotherapy. *Psychosom. Med.* **13**, 82.

MURPHY, W. F. (1958). A comparison of psycho-analysis with dynamic psychotherapies. *J. nerv. ment. Dis.* **126**, 441.

NEUSTATTER, W. L. (1935). The results in fifty cases treated by psychotherapy. *Lancet, i*, 796.

OBERNDORF, C. P. (1947). Constant elements in psychotherapy. *Yearb. Psychoanal.* **3**, 175.

OBERNDORF, C. P., GREENACRE, P., and KUBIE, L. (1948). Symposium on the evaluation of therapeutic results. *Int. J. Psycho-anal.* **29**, 7.

PHILLIPS, E. L. and JOHNSTON, M. S. H. (1954). Parent-child psychotherapy. *Psychiatry*, **17**, 267.

PHILLIPSON, H. (1955). *The object relations technique.* London: Tavistock Publications.

PUMPIAN-MINDLIN, E. (1953). Considerations in the selection of patients for short-term therapy. *Amer. J. Psychother.* **7**, 641.

RIPLEY, H., WOLF, S., and WOLFF, H. (1948). Treatment in a psychosomatic clinic. *J. Amer. med. Ass.* **138**, 949.

ROGERS, C. R. (1951). *Client-centered therapy.* New York: Houghton Mifflin Co.

ROGERS, C. R. and Dymond, F. (1954). *Psychotherapy and personality change.* Chicago: University of Chicago Press.

ROSENBAUM, M., FRIEDLANDER, J., and KAPLAN, S. M. (1956). Evaluation of the results of psychotherapy. *Psychosom. Med.* **18**, 113.

ROTHENBERG, S. (1955). Brief psychodynamically oriented therapy. *Psychosom. Med.* **17**, 455.

SASLOW, G. and PETERS, A. (1956). A follow-up study of 'untreated' patients with various behaviour disorders. *Psychiat. Quart.* **30**, 283.

References

SAUL, L. J. (1951). On the value of one or two interviews. *Psychoanal. Quart.* **20**, 613.

SCHJELDERUP, H. (1936). Charakterveränderungen durch psychoanalytische Behandlung. *Acta Psychiat. Kbh.* **11**, 631.

SCHJELDERUP, H. (1955). Lasting effects of psycho-analytic treatment. *Psychiatry*, **18**, 109.

SEITZ, P. F. D. (1953). Dynamically oriented brief psychotherapy in psycho-cutaneous excoriation syndromes. *Psychosom. Med.* **15**, 200.

SIMPSON, S. L. (1959). *Major endocrine disorders.* London: Oxford University Press.

STEKEL, W. (1911), Über ein Zeremoniell vor dem Schlafengehen. *Zbl. Psychoan.* **2**, 557.

STEKEL, W. (1923). *Zwang und Zweifel.* Berlin, Vienna: Urban und Schwarzenberg. English translation by E. Gutheil: *Compulsion and doubt.* New York: Liveright Publishing Corp. (1949).

STEKEL, W. (1938). *Technik der analytischen Psychotherapie.* Berne: Medizinischer Verlag Hans Huber. English translation by Eden and Cedar Paul: *Technique of analytical psychotherapy.* London: Bodley Head (1950).

STONE, L. (1951). Psychoanalysis and brief psychotherapy. *Psychoanal. Quart.* **20**, 215.

STRUPP, H. H. (1960). *Psychotherapists in action.* New York: Grune and Stratton.

SULLIVAN, P. L., MILLER, C., and SMELSER, W. (1958). Factors in length of stay and progress in psychotherapy. *J. cons. Psychol.* **22**, 1.

TANNENBAUM, S. A. (1913). Über einen durch Psychoanalyse geheilten Fall von Dyspareunie. *Zbl. Psychoan.* **4**, 373.

TEUBER, H. L. and POWERS, E. (1953). Evaluating therapy in a delinquency prevention program. *Res. Publ. Ass. nerv. ment. Dis.* **31**, 138.

THOMPSON, CLARA (1952). *Psychoanalysis, evolution and development.* London: George Allen & Unwin; New York: Hermitage House (1950).

THORNE, F. C. (1957). An evaluation of eclectically oriented psychotherapy. *J. cons. Psychol.* **21**, 459.

VOSBURG, R. L. (1958). Some remarks on psychotherapy as reflected in hospital charts. *Psychiatric communications of the Western Psychiatric Institute, University of Pittsburgh*, **1**, 151.

WALLACE, H. E. R. and WHYTE, M. B. H. (1959). Natural history of the psychoneuroses. *Brit. med. J.* **i**, 144.

WATTERSON, D. J. (1960). Reflections on the progress of psychotherapy. In *Panel on brief psychotherapy. Canadian Psychiatric Ass. J.* **5**, 166.

WINDLE, C. (1952). Psychological tests in psychopathological prognosis. *Psychol. Bull.* **49**, 451.

WOLPE, J. (1958). *Psychotherapy by reciprocal inhibition.* California: Stanford University Press.

WULFF, M. (1910). Zur Psychologie der 'Schwangenschaftsneurose'. *Zbl. Psychoan.* **1**, 339.

YASKIN, J. C. (1936). The psychoneuroses and neuroses. A review of a hundred cases with special reference to treatment and results. *Amer. J. Psychiat.* **93**, 107.

Index

Index

Index

Oberndorf, C. P.
see also Obendorf, Greenacre & Kubie
long follow-up of early psychoanalyses, 10
Oberndorf, C. P., Greenacre, P. & Kubie, L.
see also Bandler
case history of Bandler's, 23
object relations, *see* human relations; personal relations
Object Relations Test (ORT), use of, in present work, 40
'objective' methods
in assessment of therapeutic results
Rogers & Dymond, 154
Teuber & Powers, 152
disadvantages of, 4
in handling of clinical judgements, 270–1
limitations of, 48
in present work, 5, 233–72
'Oedipal' problems
hypothesis of good prognosis in, 178
outcome in, 182
one-tailed test, meaning of, 173 (fn)
'oral' disposition, a contra-indication to brief psychotherapy (Berliner), 18 (table)
'oral' material contra-indicated in brief psychotherapy (Fuerst), 30
'oral' problems, hypothesis of poor prognosis in, 178
ORT, use of, in present work, 40
outcome of therapy
see also therapeutic results
list of scores for, 171
and various factors in patient and in therapy, e.g. motivation, transference interpretation, etc., *see* motivation; transference interpretation, etc.
over-determination, a lengthening factor, 7, 281
attempt to overcome, by focal technique, 210
'own controls', in the study of Rogers & Dymond, 153–4

P ratio, *see* parent ratio
palaeontology, observations not always repeatable, 269
palliative nature of brief psychotherapy (Rado), 22, 170
contradicted in present work, 170
parallel variation, hypothesis of, *see* hypothesis

Paranoid Engineer, the, a patient in the present work
absence of projection test in, 40
Assessment and Therapy Form, 104–6
and dependence, 231
disturbing interpretations in, 203
failure to terminate in, 231, 264
motivation, 197–8
psychopathology
in relation to outcome, 181
in relation to selection, 180
result of long-term therapy in, 197–8
a severely ill patient in present work, 180, 181, 197–8
time limit in, 209
traumatic memory in, 213
parent
see also parent-oriented therapies; parent ratio
interpretations directed towards, 237
link with therapist, *see* therapist-parent link
parent-oriented therapies, and outcome, 244–5 (table), 248
parent ratio, and outcome, 244–5 (table), 248
partial interpretations
see also trial interpretations
use of, in present work, 203–4
partial resolution, definition of, 47
passivity, in therapist, a lengthening factor, 7, 8, 281
attempt to overcome, by focal technique, 210
avoidance of, in brief psychotherapy, 28–9
opposed by Ferenczi, 13–14
past experiences
see also childhood; therapist-parent link
link with transference and life situation (Glover, Alexander), 250–1
pathological process, in medical and psychodynamic diagnosis, 44
patients in the present study,
characteristics of, 179–80, 273
individual, *see* individual pseudonyms
selection of, etc., *see* selection, etc.
perfectionism, therapeutic, a lengthening factor,
avoidance of, 28–9, 281
Pumpian-Mindlin on, 29
'person', towards whom interpretations are directed, 236–7, 243–6
personal relations, history of, a selection criterion

Index

304

311

Index